CT of the Retroperitoneum

Giorgio Ascenti · Angelo Vanzulli
Carlo Catalano · Rendon C. Nelson

CT of the Retroperitoneum

From Conventional to Multi-energy Imaging

Springer

Giorgio Ascenti
Department of Biomedical Sciences
and Morphological and Functional
Imaging
University of Messina
Messina
Italy

Angelo Vanzulli
Department of Radiology
Niguarda General Hospital
Milan
Italy

Carlo Catalano
Department of Radiological,
Oncological and Pathological Sciences
Sapienza University of Rome
Rome
Italy

Rendon C. Nelson
Department of Radiology
Duke University Medical Center
Durham
USA

ISBN 978-88-470-5879-8 ISBN 978-88-470-5469-1 (eBook)
DOI 10.1007/978-88-470-5469-1
Springer Milan Heidelberg New York Dordrecht London

Printed on acid-free paper

Springer is part of Springer Science+Business Media (www.springer.com)

Foreword

For a long time, retroperitoneal organs and its associated myriad of abnormalities represented a "sanctuary of inaccessibility" for early medical imaging, with the pathologists being the only umpire in these scenarios.

With early detection and precise disease characterization, the advent of CT first, and then multidetector CT—with isotropic voxel technology— has represented the transition from black-and-white to colors for a number of retroperitoneal affections. Over the subsequent years, the radiologists' community has assisted to a sprout of innovations which has, more recently, led to dual energy CT with multi-energy applications.

The editors of this volume, experts of high international profile in the field of abdominal imaging and, particularly, in Dual Energy CT applications, have to be commended for their outstanding job and for realizing an up-to-date guide to the use of most recent advances in multi-energy imaging.

It is with enormous pleasure I "lead off the dancing" to this volume which, I am confident, will spark fervid interest of readers to new MDCT approaches in retroperitoneal disease.

Prof. Antonio Rotondo
(Chief of the Chair of Radiology at the Second
University of Naples "Department of Clinical
and Experimental Internal Medicine,
F. Magrassi–A. Lanzara")
Chief of the I/II Department of Radiology at the
University Hospital Second University of Naples
Naples, Italy

Preface

The transition from single-detector to multidetector row CT (MDCT) in the early 2000s has dramatically changed the imaging approach to abdominal organs. MDCT implies the simultaneous activation of multiple detector rows arranged along the z-axis with acquisition of interweaving helical sections. By exploiting the increased coverage along the z-axis and taking full advantage of the rapid image acquisition, body MDCT imaging relies on scanning the abdominal viscera with a multiphasic approach, before and after contrast medium administration. In particular, timing of the contrast medium bolus can be optimized for accomplishing different diagnostic abdominal tasks, including a synchronous assessment of vascular and parenchymal compartments.

The need for protocol optimization, controlling radiation exposure to patients, and managing the large amount of data generated, represent the other side of the coin of MDCT with which the body radiologist has to face and needs to be sensitized. However the constraint to a merely attenuation-based approach represents the main drawback of modern MDCT imaging which does not exceed calculation of materials linear attenuation coefficients in Hounsfield Units (HU).

By obtaining data at different photon energies and, thereby detecting differences in material composition based on differences in photon absorption, dual energy CT recently raised to prime time for its numerous applications in body imaging. Although this technique had been already investigated in the late 1970s, owing to limitations of early prototypes (eg., the need for two separate scans with consequent radiation dose increase and image misregistration) dual energy CT has been pushed aside.

Tremendous efforts scanner manufacturers have devoted towards the development of new hardware and software strategies, as well as a growing interest in the scientific imaging community have led to an impressive expansion of dual energy CT technology which is no longer confined to a few academic institutions. As opposed to conventional MDCT imaging, dual-energy CT may represent a paradigm-shift from an attenuationbased to a material-specific quantitative approach. The general excitement for this imaging technology, however, has been paralleled by concerns about the increase in radiation exposure and costs, as well as by prejudices on a presumptive complexity of its applications. An overall streamlining of dual energy CT workflow and a substantial reduction of the costs represent future directions for moving forward.

The objective of this volume is to provide the reader with an overview of conventional MDCT approach for retroperitoneal organs, as well as to show, in the same clinical scenarios, how dual energy and multi energy CT applications can enhance the diagnoses of retroperitoneal diseases.

Prof. Giorgio Ascenti

Contents

Contributors

Diana Artioli Department of Radiology, Niguarda General Hospital, Milan, Italy

Giorgio Ascenti Department of Biomedical Sciences and Morphological and Functional Imaging, University of Messina, Policlinico "G. Martino", Messina, Italy

Alfredo Blandino Department of Biomedical Sciences and Morphological and Functional Imaging, University of Messina, Policlinico "G. Martino", Messina, Italy

Carlo Catalano Department of Radiological, Oncological and Pathological Sciences, Sapienza University of Rome, Rome, Italy

Daniel Geiger Department of Radiological, Oncological and Pathological Sciences, Sapienza University of Rome, Rome, Italy

Lisa M. Ho Department of Radiology, Duke University Medical Center, Durham, NC, USA

Bernhard Krauss Siemens AG , Healthcare Sector, Imaging & Therapy Division, Forchheim, Germany

Daniele Marin Department of Radiology, Duke University Medical Center, Durham, NC, USA

Silvio Mazziotti Department of Biomedical Sciences and Morphological and Functional Imaging, University of Messina, Policlinico "G. Martino", Messina, Italy

Achille Mileto Department of Biomedical Sciences and Morphological and Functional Imaging, University of Messina, Policlinico "G. Martino", Messina, ItalyDepartment of Radiology, Duke University Medical Center, Durham, NC, USA

Rendon C. Nelson Department of Radiology, Duke University Medical Center, Durham, NC, USA

Emanuele Scribano Department of Biomedical Sciences and Morphological and Functional Imaging, University of Messina, Policlinico "G. Martino", Messina, Italy

Carmelo Sofia Department of Biomedical Sciences and Morphological and Functional Imaging, University of Messina, Policlinico "G. Martino", Messina, Italy

Angelo Vanzulli Department of Radiology, Niguarda General Hospital, Milan, Italy

Introduction and Technical Principles 1

Angelo Vanzulli and Diana Artioli

Technological advances continuously increase the clinical applications and diagnostic value of CT.

CT was born in the late 1960s, and spiral CT was introduced just in the early 1990s; it marked one of the important steps in the evolution of CT imaging techniques. This technology allowed to acquire volume data without the risk of miss- or double-registration, enabling the reconstruction of images at any position along the patient's length axis as well as reconstructions of overlapping images to improve the longitudinal resolution. It also reduced scan times significantly.

The introduction of multi-detector row computed tomography in 1998 (MDCT) allowed other improvements. Larger anatomical volumes could be acquired with a single acquisition. The first generation of MDCT systems offered simultaneous acquisition of 4 slices, which provided considerably improved scan speed and longitudinal resolution as well as better utilization of the available X-ray power. MDCT also made longer scan ranges with substantially reduced slice width feasible, which is essential, for example, in CT angiography. The introduction of 16-slice CT scanner enabled isotropic sub-millimeter spatial resolution.

The generation of 64-slice CT systems was introduced in 2004. Two different technologies were launched in the market.

Scanners introduced by GE, Philips, and Toshiba increased the volume coverage speed by using 64 detector rows instead of 16, with a body coverage along the Z-axis of about 4 cm. Scanner introduced by Siemens used 32 physical detector rows (body coverage about 2 cm) in combination with "double Z sampling," enabled by periodically moving the focal point in the *Z* direction, in order to simultaneously acquire 64 overlapping slices. The objective of this system was to increase the longitudinal resolution and reduce spiral artifacts independent of pitch. Acquisition is faster with 64 detector rows but *Z*-axis resolution is more accurate with double *Z* sampling (0.38-mm instead of 0.6 mm).

A recent development in CT has been the introduction of dual-energy technology (2005). Dual-energy CT implies simultaneously acquiring data sets at two different photon spectra [1].

Dual-energy CT is limited to two energies. Multi-energy imaging is a challenge today and has the potential to greatly expand the clinical application of tissue differentiation.

In this chapter, technical aspects of dual- and multi-energy CT will be analyzed.

1.1 Dual-Energy CT

The first experiments with dual-energy CT date back to the late 1970s. However, the poor spatial resolution of early computed tomography and the long scan durations at that time prevented the application of the technique. Another major problem was that tube technology did not provide sufficient tube currents at low tube voltages to achieve a sufficient output of quanta relative to the higher voltage tube. Dual-energy

G. Ascenti et al., *CT of the Retroperitoneum*,
DOI: 10.1007/978-88-470-5469-1_1, © Springer-Verlag Italia 2014

technology aims to better distinguish different materials in body tissues, thus improving diagnostic power of CT.

Recently, three dual-energy CT systems have been developed and are commercially available: Dual Source, Rapid kV switching, Sequential Dual Energy [2]. Regardless the kind of CT system, material differentiation is based on the same physical X-rays interactions with materials.

The differentiation of material in computed tomography is based on their X-ray attenuation as quantified in Hounsfield Units and displayed in shades of gray at different window levels in normal CT scans. Attenuation is caused by absorption and scattering of radiation by the material under investigation. The two main mechanisms responsible for these effects in the photon energy range used in CT are the Compton scatter and the photoelectric effect.

Photoelectric effect is produced when a low-energy photon collides with an electron; the energy is completely absorbed by the electron, which moves from its position; an ionized atom is obtained and the photon disappears.

Compton effect is produced when a high-energy photon collides with an electron. In this case, the electron absorbs a part of the energy and moves inducing an ionized atom; a new photon, with lower energy and a different direction, is emitted. If the scattered photon still has enough energy left, the process may be repeated (Fig. 1.1).

Another important physical phenomenon should be taken into account while thinking of X-rays interactions: k edge.

K edge describes a sudden increase in the attenuation coefficient of photons occurring at a photon energy just above the binding energy of the K shell electron of the atoms interacting with the photons. The sudden increase in attenuation is due to photoelectric absorption of the photons. For this interaction to occur, the photons must have more energy than the binding energy of the K-shell electrons. A photon having an energy just above the binding energy of the electron is therefore more likely to be absorbed than a photon having an energy just below this binding energy.

The two X-ray contrast media iodine and barium have ideal K-shell binding energies for absorption of X-rays, 33.2 and 37.4 keV, respectively, which is close to the mean energy of most diagnostic X-ray beams.

X-ray absorption depends on the inner electron shells: dual-energy CT is sensitive to atomic number and density, but it is not sensitive to chemical binding.

Considering that any substance has a different photoelectric effect, Compton effect and k-edge at different energy levels, it is possible to understand how dual-energy CT works.

In particular at 80 kV, iodine has its maximum absorption; applying different X-ray spectra and analyzing the differences in attenuation, as we can see in dual-energy acquisition, iodine can be easily differentiated from other materials that do not show its behavior at 80 kV. Iodine is the unique material that doubles its HU values from 140 to 80 kV. At 80 kV, some other materials have higher CT values such as bone, metal, but do not double; at 140 kV, some materials have higher CT values, such as fat, plastic, uric acid; moreover, some materials have the same CT values at 80 and 140 kV, such as water, soft tissues, blood. Since these material behavior is known, tissues can be differentiated [3].

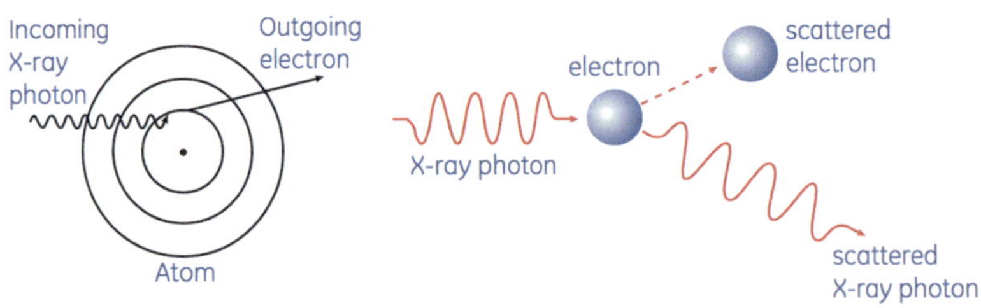

Fig. 1.1 Photoelectric effect (*left*) and compton effect (*right*) are the physical basis of X-ray attenuation (Courtesy of GE Healthcare, Waukesha, U.S.A.)

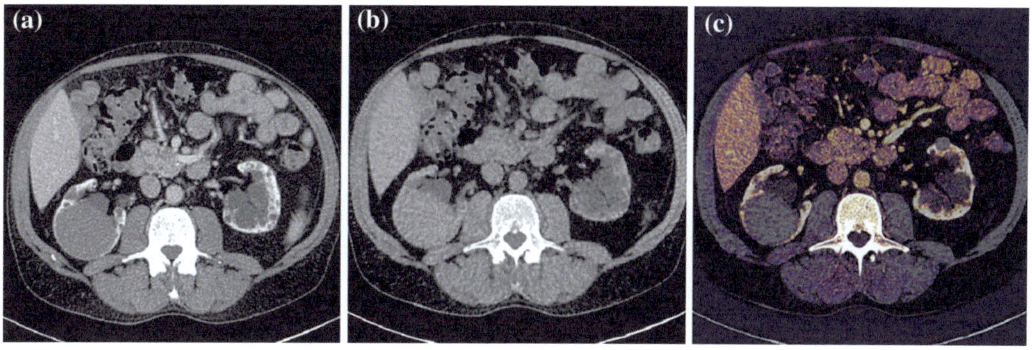

Fig. 1.2 An hyperdense mass can be seen in the diagnostic image (**a**), in the Virtual Non-Contrast (VNC) image (**b**), obtained with subtraction of iodine data, the mass results already hyperdense without contrast; moreover, in iodine map image (**c**) the mass has not iodine enhancement. Therefore, in a single dual-energy acquisition, the diagnosis can be obtained (hyperdense cyst. Courtesy of Siemens AG, Muenchen, Germany)

Considering iodine properties at 80 kV, in dual-energy CT a virtual-unenhanced image can be generated, and this data may be used for baseline density measurements, thereby making true unenhanced imaging unnecessary and saving radiation.

Using dual-energy post-processing software, the contrast agent can be digitally subtracted from the image. This can be done because the dual-energy index of iodine is significantly different from the dual-energy index of soft tissue and fat. The dual-energy data can also be used to generate a color-coded image that shows the distribution of iodine within the volume of tissue examined by CT. This color-coded display is very sensitive to subtle enhancement.

In abdominal imaging, for example, this can be useful in cases of incidentally detected renal lesions with high attenuation on unenhanced CT, the main differential diagnostic considerations being hyperdense cysts and renal masses (Fig. 1.2).

Immediately after reconstruction, the images can be semi-automatically post-processed, offering the radiologist a fast diagnosis.

In clinical application, dual energy helps to visualize and segmentate vessels, contrast media, tendons, ligaments, kidney stones, gout deposits, perfused blood volume, hard plaque, iodine content in small vessels. Any of these structure often has its dedicated software application for analysis. Moreover, post-processing applications can give additional information about body tissues composition.

Groups of two or three materials are usually analyzed; for example, iodine, soft tissue, and water, or water, calcium, and uric acid (kidney stones application); for the visualization of calcifications in the setting of a contrast-enhanced examination, the algorithm will analyze iodine, calcium, and soft-tissue densities [4].

1.2 Dual-Source CT

In dual-source CT system, released by Siemens in 2005, two X-ray tubes with two corresponding detectors are mounted onto a rotating gantry with a 90 angular offset (Fig. 1.3).

For each tube, a 64-slice design (Siemens Somatom Definition) is present: the "A" detector, which is equal in size to a standard detector (50 cm), and the "B" detector, which also has a 64-slice design, but with a reduced field of view of 27 cm. This detector array provides high spatial resolution of isotropic 0.38 mm edge-length voxels and allows a rapid acquisition of a *Z*-axis volume.

In 2008, the second-generation DSCT "Siemens Somatom Definition Flash" was introduced. It features even faster gantry rotation (0.28 s), twice the number of detector slices and a larger field of view (332 mm) [5].

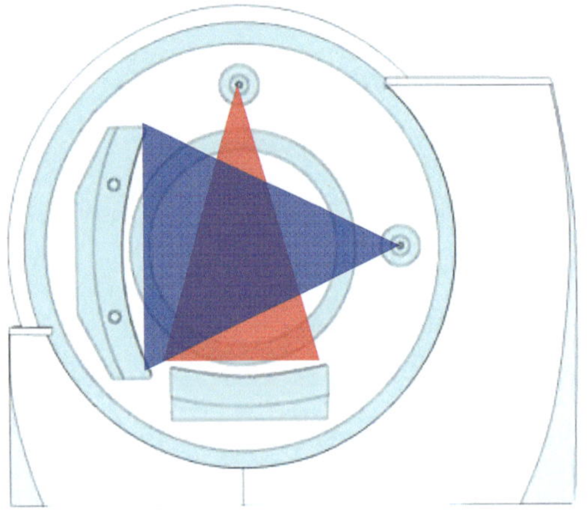

Fig. 1.3 Geometry of dual-source CT (Courtesy of Siemens AG, Muenchen, Germany)

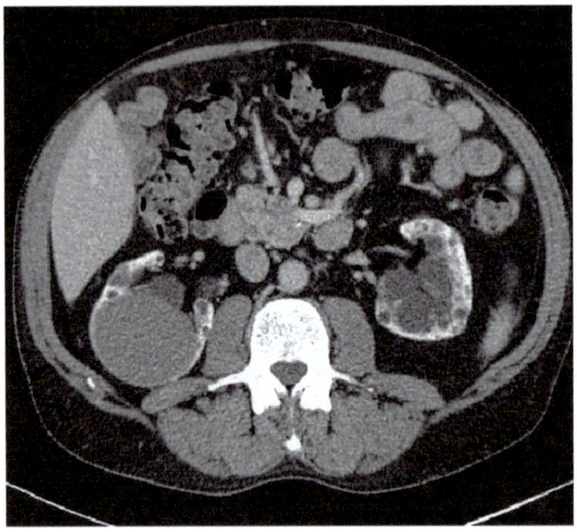

Fig. 1.4 Example of a mixed 140–80 kV image, resulting in a common 120 kV diagnostic image (Courtesy of Siemens AG, Muenchen, Germany)

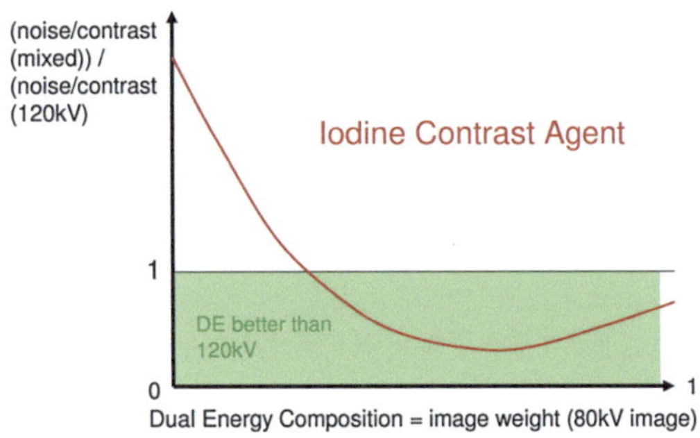

Fig. 1.5 When the contribution of 80 kV data in mixed images is correct (*left part*), high response of iodine to 80 kV tube current leads to better contrast to noise ratio than simple 120 kV standard images (Courtesy of Siemens AG, Muenchen, Germany)

This CT system allows almost simultaneous acquisition of two energy data sets, with very few artifacts due to image misregistration.

The acquired projection data primarily have to be reconstructed by standard filtered back-projection, separately for the two simultaneously acquired spiral data sets (80 and 140 kV). Subsequently, materials can be analyzed; this data analysis is called post-reconstruction analysis, meaning that different materials are analyzed after standard reconstruction for each tube. This system differs from material decomposition obtained by GE.

For abdominal imaging, dual-energy CT acquisitions should employ a collimation of 14 × 1.2 mm rather than 64 × 0.6 mm as the latter configuration will cause increased image noise on the B detector images. Since a reconstructed slice thickness below 1.2 mm is usually not required for most applications in the abdomen, this typically does not represent a significant limitation in terms of spatial resolution. However, the data acquired are not isotropic.

Each dual-energy acquisition can generate the following types of data: pure 80 kVp data, pure 140 kVp data, and a weighted average 120 kVp data set that usually is a composition of 70 % from the A (high kV) and 30 % from the B (low kV) tube (Fig. 1.4). This relation can be manually adjusted on a dual-energy workstation.

Note that at same dose a dual energy mixed image has better contrast/noise ratio than 120 kV routine images, due to the contribution of 80 kV data, where the absorption peak of iodine is at its maximum (Fig. 1.5) [3].

Dual-source CT, when compared with a single-source system, presents two other possible applications. First, the tubes can be used at equal tube potentials, permitting increased photon flux in larger patients. Second, since an image can be acquired using 2 × 90 degrees of gantry rotation rather than 180, temporal resolution can be increased by a factor of two when using the two tubes at identical kVp levels [4]. Using this technique, a temporal resolution of 70 ms is possible; this is most useful for cardiac imaging.

1.3 Dose

To minimize patient exposure to ionizing radiation, abdominal dual-energy CT protocols operate using an online dose modulation system (CareDOSE 4D, Siemens) that adapts the tube current to the patient's anatomy [6]. The image quality reference mAs values are usually set to 400 mAs on the B tube and 96 mAs on the A tube, thereby splitting the energy between the two tubes. These settings take into account that higher mAs values on the A tube would lead to increased image noise on the B detector due to scatter radiation. The calculated effective patient doses for abdominal scans will range from 4.5–12.5 mSv, which is similar to the effective dose of a standard abdominal CT acquisition using 120 kVp with 250 mAs [4].

Dual-energy CT is not recommended for patients whose body mass index is >30. In morbidly obese patients, the two tubes can both be operated at 120 kVp, which will help to decrease image noise in these very large patients. The system can be used to scan patients with a body weight of up to 500 lbs (220 kg).

1.4 Limitations

A limitation of first-generation dual-source CT in the abdomen and pelvis is that the smaller size of the B detector will prevent imaging of the entire FOV in larger patients. Therefore, patients may have to be positioned off center if the location of the lesion is in the periphery of the FOV (for example renal masses). Therefore, it is mandatory to acquire two topograms. Moreover, objects at the outer periphery of the B detector may be unable to undergo optimal post-processing due to the technical specifications of the post-processing algorithm. In detail, adjacent voxels have to be used for calculation of the DE properties of any voxel within the field of view. The reconstructed DE field of view is 5 mm smaller than the actual B detector FOV.

Grosjean et al. have reported a significant impairment of the efficiency of DE analysis by motion during CT [7]. Thus, they conclude a perfect breath-hold during CT is essential [8].

1.5 Rapid kVp Switching or Gemstone Spectral Imaging

The CT system released by GE is a single X-ray source system that employs fast kVp switching for dual-energy acquisitions. It is called Gemstone spectral imaging (GSI), and it is based on projection-based material decomposition.

This technique enables precise temporal registration of views, freezing motion as the alternating spectrums penetrate the patient, thereby significantly reducing motion artifacts.

The generator and tube are capable of reliably switching between 80 and 140 kVp targets and have the capability to support sampling as quickly as every 140 microseconds.

The Gemstone detector is a key contributor to fast kVp switching acquisitions through its scintillator and data acquisition system (DAS). It is a complex rare earth based oxide, which has a chemically replicated garnet crystal structure. This lends itself to imaging that requires high light output, fast primary speed, very low afterglow, and almost undetectable radiation damage. Gemstone has a primary decay time of only 30 ns, making it 100 times faster than GOS (Gd2O2S), while also having afterglow levels that reach only 25 % of GOS levels making it ideal for fast sampling. The capabilities of the scintillator are matched with a fast sampling capability DAS, enabling simultaneous acquisition of low and high kVp sinograms.

In order to combat the traditional flux issues that have challenged fast kV switching, low-kVp and high-kVp acquisitions are flux balanced through advances in the DAS, which allow for dynamically changing view integration times. Additional time is allocated to the low-kVp acquisition relative to the high-kV acquisition in order to reduce photon starvation conditions.

Coupled with the appropriate rotation speed, a more balanced flux condition between the two kVp scans is achieved and serves to minimize patient dose.

1.6 Reconstruction

The overall spectrum is decomposed into a superposition of several known kVp spectra through the measurement of the detector response to attenuation.

Once a GSI acquisition is completed, the imaging reconstruction/processing chain, in combination with the GSI viewer, provides the user different kinds of images, such as conventional low-/high-kVp Hounsfield (HU) attenuation, material density and monochromatic keV HU representations of the data.

We commonly define the X-ray beam quality in terms of kVp (kilovoltage peak) denoting the maximum photon energy, since the X-ray beam is comprised of a mixture of X-ray photon energies (Fig. 1.6).

If we measure the X-ray attenuation of an object at two different spectrums, low kVp and high kVp, we can mathematically transform the attenuation measurements into the density of two materials that would be needed to produce the measured attenuation. This process is referred to as material decomposition or material separation.

Material decomposition does not identify materials. Rather, given two selected basis materials, material decomposition determines how much of each material would be needed to produce the observed low- and high-kVp measurements. Generally, low- and high-attenuating materials are selected as the basis pair. For diagnostic imaging, water and iodine are often used, since they span the atomic number range of materials generally found in medical imaging and approximate soft tissue and iodinated contrast, resulting in material density images that are intuitive to interpret.

Monochromatic images may be synthesized from the material density images. The monochromatic image depicts how the imaged object would look if the X-ray source produced only X-ray photons at a single energy. Through this calculation, material decomposition enables the representation of the data as though it came from a monochromatic source. Monochromatic images are free of beam hardening and are a significant step toward quantitative imaging. These images remain subject to errors induced by scatter, aliasing and partial volume. Generally, the monochromatic image is similar to that of a conventional HU image with fewer artifacts. The monochromatic energy is selectable with higher energies yielding less contrast between materials and more contrast with low energies. GSI viewer enables selection of 101 keV energy levels virtual images (Figs. 1.7 and 1.8) [9].

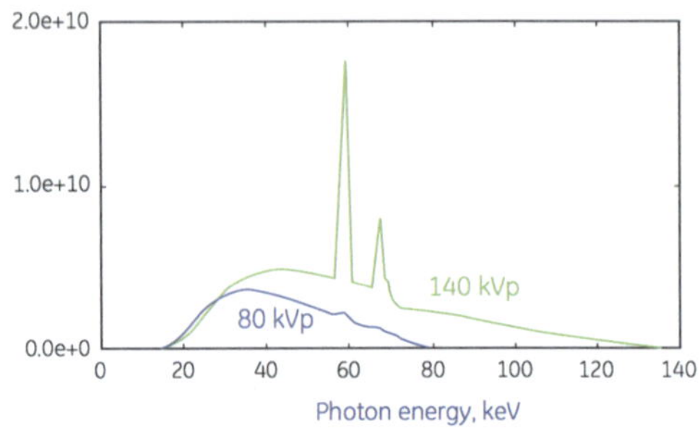

Fig. 1.6 Polychromatic X-ray spectrums for 80 and 140 kVp (Courtesy of GE Healthcare, Waukesha, U.S.A.)

1.7 Sequential Dual Energy

Sequential Dual Energy (SDE) released by Philips is a technique using two consecutive scans with different energies (iCT version 3.2). Technological requirements are more simple for this kind of acquisition, compared with Dual Source and GSI.

There are no factory default scanning protocols for Sequential Dual Energy; the user should create a tailored protocol; a dedicated software is available for reconstructions (EBW Spectral Analysis). Protocols include two Coupled Acquisitions with a minimal delay between them (Currently 2.1 s). There is a single axial rotation (<=8 cm coverage), without couch movement; there must be identical scan Length, FOV and scan parameters except for kV and mAs. Any

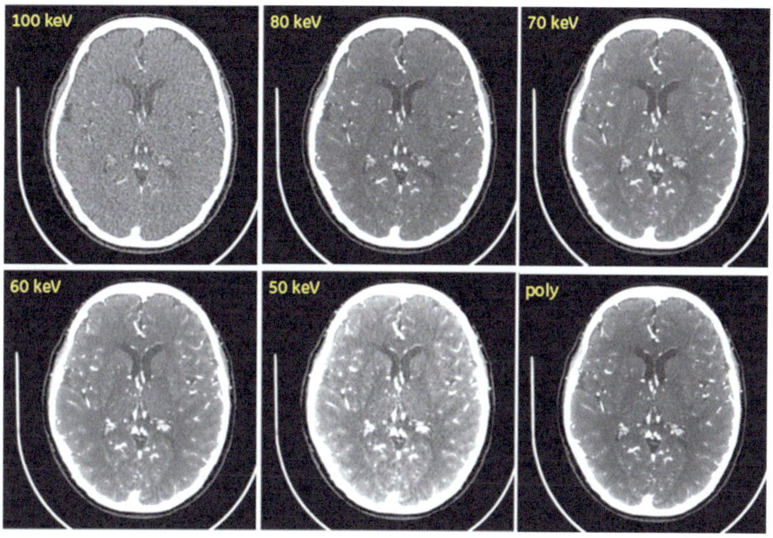

Fig. 1.7 Monochromatic renderings of a head image. Changes in noise and contrast can be seen (Courtesy of GE Healthcare, Waukesha, U.S.A.)

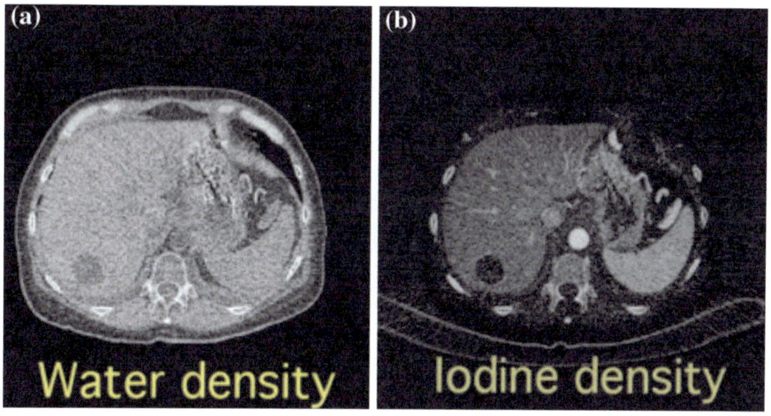

Fig. 1.8 Example of material decomposition with water (**a**) and iodine (**b**) images (Courtesy of GE Healthcare, Waukesha, U.S.A.)

two kV can be selected for SDE, but the best tissue differentiation can be achieved with a large kV difference (i.e., 140 and 80 kV), as well as for Dual Source and GSI. In order to have same image quality despite differences in kV, CTDI ratio should be 1; that means higher mAs with lower kV. After acquisition, the two scans must be aligned before analysis. A virtual mean kV image can be easily obtained from the two series. The workstation starts the analysis computing pixel values. Each pixel has two different values at high and low energy; the ratio of the two values corresponds to a specific material in an energy map.

These dual-energy series are easily achievable without a technological expense; they are also easily clinically feasible; but compared with Dual Source and GSI, they have some limitations: they are more subject to motion artifacts and can suffer from different iodine distribution at different time acquisition.

Philips implemented another experimental dual-energy system: a dual-layer detector scanner. In a single source, dual-layer detector scanner configuration, one X-ray tube is used to expose a detector consisting of two layers of scintillators. The two layers are directly on top of one another, and CT scan is performed at a high kVp. The first layer encountered by the X-ray photons absorbs most of the low-energy spectrum (approximately 50 % of the beam), while the bottom detector layer absorbs the remaining high-energy photons. Images are reconstructed separately from the data of the upper and lower layers. Since the spectral energy separation is intrinsic to the detection System, this approach eliminates the time lag of sequential techniques, making it ideal for imaging moving organs.

As in Dual Source and GSI systems, low- and high-energy images, water–iodine images can be easily obtained from data sets.

1.8 Multi-Energy CT

Multi-energy CT is not clinically applied yet, but there are some research studies giving interesting results.

In contrast to the scintillator detectors used in conventional and dual-energy CT systems, whose signal output is almost exclusively dependent on the energy flux integrated over the entire X-ray spectrum, spectral CT is based on new detector designs that may possess energy-sensitive photon-counting capability. This system allows the compartmentalization of detected X-ray photons into energy bins. Soft-tissue characterization and selective contrast material detection are subsequently achieved by recognizing tissue- and material-specific energy distributions [10].

As said before, the attenuation of X-rays is energy dependent and each substance has a specific attenuation curve [11]. Tissue characterization using X-ray is possible provided the absorption characteristics can be either measured or differentiated [12].

In dual-energy CT, materials can be differentiated by exposing the tissue to two different X-ray spectra or using a combination detector with two different energy ranges.

The disadvantages of this technique are that materials with similar attenuation curves such as iodine and barium cannot be distinguished, due to partially overlapping spectra [12].

In spectral CT imaging, a fixed broad spectrum X-ray source is used (such as used in conventional CT) combined with an energy discriminating detector that can differentiate the attenuation spectrum of all materials within the voxel [13, 14].

New developments in direct-conversion semiconductor detectors based on CZT (Cadmium–Zinc–Telluride) or CdTe (Cadmium Telluride) may enable the application of this technique also for medical CT imaging.

A prerequisite for the spectral analysis is the knowledge of the spectral response of the detector.

X-ray detector is operated in photon-counting mode applying energy discrimination by threshold values for each individual pixel. Physically, the thresholds are realized by voltages that are fed into the pulse-height comparator circuits. The pulse height obtained from the detector is nearly proportional to the energy of the detected photon, but gain and offset vary from bin to bin and from pixel to pixel. Therefore, the relationship between the measured photon energy in keV and the threshold voltage (in mV), which triggers the corresponding event, had to be determined through a calibration process.

As reported by Anderson et al. the photon-counting Medipix2 [15] and Medipix3 [16] detectors developed by the European Centre for Nuclear Research (CERN) allow up to eight points of an attenuation spectrum to be reconstructed from a single exposure without overlap in the measurement.

Other research studies are conducted by Philips [17]. Spectral CT imaging is performed with an experimental single-section CT scanner (Multi-Energy Philips Photon-Counting CT; Research Europe) that allows differentiation of detected X-ray photons into six distinct energy bins . The X-ray beam passes through the beryllium exit window of the X-ray tube and enters the detector through a 2-mm aluminum window; no further spectral filtering is applied. The photon-counting detector is based on a cadmium telluride array (MEXC; Gamma Medica Ideas, Northridge, Calif) that allows the simultaneous differentiation of detected X-ray photons according to their individual energy levels by separating the X-ray photons into six energy bins at 25–34, 34–39, 39–44, 45–49, 49–55, and more than 55 keV. These threshold levels are set prior to the initiation of spectral

CT imaging. The energy separation is not sharply delineated; instead, a smooth transition between the energy bands exists. Gantry rotation time is 120 s because of the count rate limitations of the detector system and the need to enable good photon statistics (approximately 2,000 projections per gantry revolution). For each energy bin, 0.5-mm axial sections with a matrix of 512 × 512 pixels within a 20-mm field of view are reconstructed without the additional application of reconstruction filters. The attenuation units attained with this prototype spectral CT scanner are all calibrated with a water phantom as fixed, meaning, however (in contrast to clinical Hounsfield units), that they are directly dependent on detector counts [17].

In the absence of K-edge discontinuities, the energy dependence of the linear attenuation coefficient of materials of diagnostic interest can be described accurately by a linear combination of the photo-electric and the Compton effects.

In the presence of elements with a high atomic number Z, the description of the attenuation properties of matter has to be modified. In order to correctly describe the attenuation of a sample containing a single element with K-edge discontinuity inside the relevant energy range, the decomposition has to be extended by the energy dependent attenuation function of this particular element as a third component.

In order to observe the K-edge discontinuity, it is important that the transmission spectrum provides sufficient power at lower as well as at higher X-ray energies. In the case of strongly attenuating objects, the effects of beam hardening will eventually remove power in the low-energy part of the spectrum to the extent that the discontinuity is no longer observable due to photon starvation.

It is possible, in principle, to detect k edges of lower *Z* elements, but it has to be considered that photon starvation is a serious problem in the low-energy range. Therefore, gadolinium (*Z* 64; k edge, 50.2 keV) is more promising as a spectrally detectable contrast agent than, for example, iodine (*Z* 53; k edge, 33.2 keV) [18].

For effective material decomposition, the energy bins used for material decomposition should be sufficiently narrow and well separated. However, when narrow bins are used, a large fraction of the detected X-ray counts is lost and statistical noise is increased. Alternatively, the X-ray spectrum can be split into a few larger bins with no gap in between and all detected X-ray photons can be used for material decomposition. However, in this case, the energy bins are too wide and not well separated, which results in suboptimal material decomposition. The above contradictory requirements can be resolved if the X-ray photons are physically removed from the regions of the energy spectrum between the energy bins. Such a selective removal can be performed using filtration of the X-ray beam by high-Z filter materials with appropriate positions of K-edge energies [14].

In conclusion, dual energy is clinically feasible and it has brought some advance in material differentiation, image quality and diagnostic confidence.

There are several research studies investigating multi-energy CT, in order to achieve detailed tissue differentiation. Maybe some of these results will be applied to routine clinical practice, improving diagnostic performance.

References

1. Seidensticker PR, Hofmann LK (2008) Dual source CT imaging. Springer
2. Karçaaltıncaba M, Aktaş A (2011) Dual-energy CT revisited with multidetector CT: review of principles and clinical applications. Diagn Interv Radiol 17(3):181–194
3. Siemens (2006) Syngo dual energy: physical background
4. Graser A, Johnson TRC, Chandarana H et al (2009) Dual energy CT: preliminary observations and potential clinical applications in the abdomen. Eur Radiol 19:13–23
5. Johnson TRC, Fink C, Schoenberg SO (2011) Dual energy in clinical practice. Springer, Berlin
6. Graser A, Wintersperger BJ, Suess C et al (2006) Dose reduction and image quality in MDCT colonography using tube current modulation. AJR Am J Roentgenol 187(3):695–701

7. Grosjean R, Sauer B, Guerra RM et al (2008) Characterization of human renal stones with MDCT: advantage of dual energy and limitations due to respiratory motion. AJR Am J Roentgenol 190(3):720–728
8. Thomas C, Patschan O, Ketelsen D et al (2009) Dual-energy CT for the characterization of urinary calculi: In vitro and in vivo evaluation of a low-dose scanning protocol. Eur Radiol 19:1553–1559
9. Langan DA (2008) Gemstone spectral imaging. GE Healthcare, Waukesha
10. Boll DT, Patil NA, Paulson EK et al (2010) Focal cystic high-attenuation lesions: characterization in renal phantom by using photon-counting spectral CT–improved differentiation of lesion composition. Radiology 254(1):270–276
11. Hubbell JH, Seltzer SM (1995) Tables of X-ray mass attenuation coefficients and mass-energy absorption coefficients. Physical Reference Data. NIST standard reference database 126. Available at http://physics.nist.gov/PhysRefData/XrayMassCoef/cover.html
12. Anderson NG, Butler AP, Scott NJ et al (2010) Spectroscopic (multi-energy) CT distinguishes iodine and barium contrast material in MICE. Eur Radiol 20(9):2126–2134
13. Schlomka JP, Roessl E, Dorscheid R et al (2008) Experimental feasibility of multi-energy photon-counting K-edge imaging in pre-clinical computed tomography. Phys Med Biol 53(15):4031–4047
14. Shikhaliev PM (2012) Photon counting spectral CT: improved material decomposition with K-edge-filtered X-rays. Phys Med Biol 57(6):1595–1615
15. Llopart X, Campbell M, Dinapoli R et al (2002) Medipix2, a 64 k pixel readout chip with 55 μm square elements working in single photon counting mode. IEEE Trans Nucl Sci NS- 49:2279
16. Ballabriga R, Campbell M, Heijne EHM et al (2007) The medipix3 prototype, a pixel readout chip working in a single photon counting mode with improved spectrometric performance. IEEE Trans Nucl Sci 54:1824
17. Roessl E, Proksa R (2007) K-edge imaging in x-ray computed tomography using multi-bin photon counting detectors. Phys Med Biol 52(15):4679–4696
18. Feuerlein S, Roessl E, Proksa R et al (2008) Multienergy photon-counting K-edge imaging: potential for improved luminal depiction in vascular imaging. Radiology 249(3):1010–1016

Dual-, Multi-, and Mono-Energy CT & Iodine: Basic Concepts and Clinical Applications

2

2.1 Introduction

Dual-energy computed tomography (DECT) is a relatively novel CT technique available in advanced diagnostic units. DECT implies the application of two different energies. It adds, to the classic single-energy multi-detector CT study, information yielded from material differentiation derived from the interaction between tissues and different energy levels [1]. Dual-energy computed tomographs exploit the two energy spectra using a dual-tube configuration working at different voltages with intersecting radiation beams or a single tube with fast voltage switching, or using energy-sensitive sandwich detectors [2, 3]. DECT is presently offered by major vendors and recently transitioned from first- to second-generation apparatuses [4]. Second-generation models overcome limitations of older scanners, such as the smaller field of view (FOV) of the lower-energy tube, in the dual-tube configuration. Dual-source approach (Siemens Healthcare, Forchheim, Germany) appears to be presently the most diffused technique, with a lesser diffusion of rapid kVp-switching (GE Milwaukee, WI) and energy-sensitive sandwich detectors (Philips, Cleveland, OH) [3].

As a matter of fact, from first experimental applications in the early 1980s, DECT has undergone major technical improvements [5, 6], proving its usefulness in abdominal [7], thoracic [8], vascular [9], orthopedic [10], and neuro [11] applications.

Multi-energy CT (*spectral imaging*) is a more specific material decomposition method. It implies material attenuation characteristics evaluation at multiple energies and in narrow ranges. The CT tube is operated using a single voltage producing a broad energy spectrum. Then, energy-sensitive detectors separate the beam into energy bands [3, 12]. This promising technique is presently under investigation and clinical applications restricted to research environments.

Aim of this chapter is to briefly draw reader's attention to the relation existing between different CT energies and iodine and how it may be exploitable in DECT. We will also briefly discuss this relation in multi-energy and mono-energetic low-kVp CT.

2.2 Basic Concepts

2.2.1 Compton, Photoelectric Effect, and the "K-edge"

The rationale behind DECT is that knowing how a substance behaves when exposed at different energies provides information about tissue composition, unobtainable with a single-energy approach [13, 14]. In spectral imaging, such analysis takes advantage of photon-counting energy-sensitive detectors [3].

In general, material attenuation is represented by a CT number (HU) related to Compton and photoelectric effect, both material and energy

G. Ascenti et al., *CT of the Retroperitoneum*,
DOI: 10.1007/978-88-470-5469-1_2, © Springer-Verlag Italia 2014

dependent. The former almost independent of photon energy, occurring at energies higher than 30 keV, related to material density. The latter predominating at lower photon energies, energy dependent, related to high atomic numbers. Different energy levels influence these two mechanisms [2] (Fig. 2.1).

Compton scattering [15] occurs when photons interact with outermost valence electrons, when the incident photon energy exceeds the binding energy of the free electron, that is ejected [16].

Photoelectric effect is the ejection of an electron from the innermost shell of an atom (K shell) by an incident photon. The void is filled from an adjacent shell causing energy release in the form of a photoelectron. The *K-shell* binding energy varies for each element and is directly proportional to the atomic number [16].

The *K-edge* is the spike in attenuation occurring at energy levels greater than that of the K-shell binding. K-edge values vary for each element and increase according to the atomic number. Photoelectric effect and K-edge behavior are the basis of DECT technique [2].

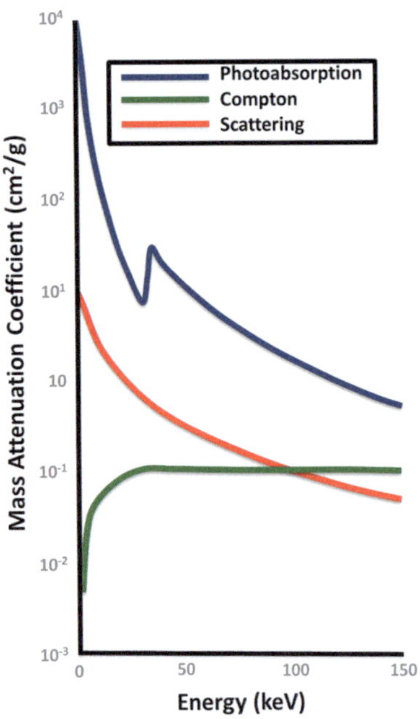

Fig. 2.1 Graph shows iodine photoabsorption (*blue*), Compton effect (*green*), and coherent (*Rayleigh*) scattering (*red*) at different energies. Note that photoabsorption effect of iodine is maximized at 50 keV (at a mean photon energy of 80 kVp). Maximum photoabsorption is shown slightly above iodine's K-edge (33 keV)

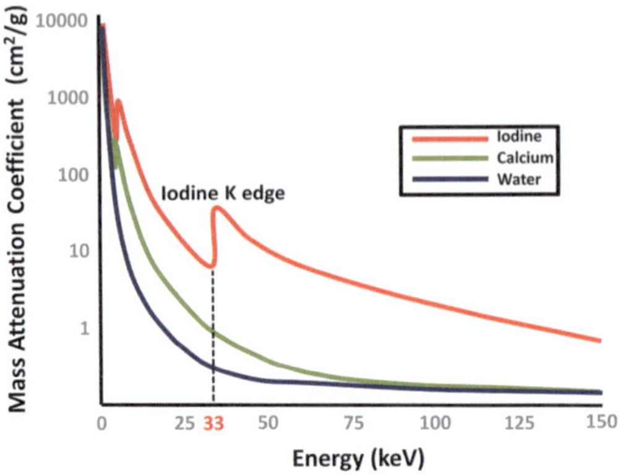

Fig. 2.2 Graph showing mass-attenuation coefficients for iodine (*red*), calcium (*green*), and water (*blue*) at different energies. Note the attenuation peak of iodine ($Z = 53$) at 33 keV

Iodine (I)-based compounds are the preferred contrast media in computed tomography. The relation between iodine ($Z = 53$) and its K-edge has been investigated [17, 18] and is set at 33 keV. The Iodine K-edge characteristics may be exploited in dual-energy and also low-kVp mono-energetic CT protocols [19–25]. The advantage is the enhanced conspicuity of iodine and a relative dose reduction. In this regard, we acknowledge that kVp and effective radiation dose share an exponential relation where mAs and dose a linear one [26]. As a drawback, a high-tube-current (mAs) setting is technically necessary to decrease image rumor [23].

Material differentiation, including iodine, derived from a multi-energy approach is at the basis of various DECT clinical applications (Fig. 2.2).

2.3 DECT and Iodinated CM in Clinical Practice

Material differentiation and contrast material quantification–identification are based upon the previously described basic technical principles, making the DECT technique highly attractive.

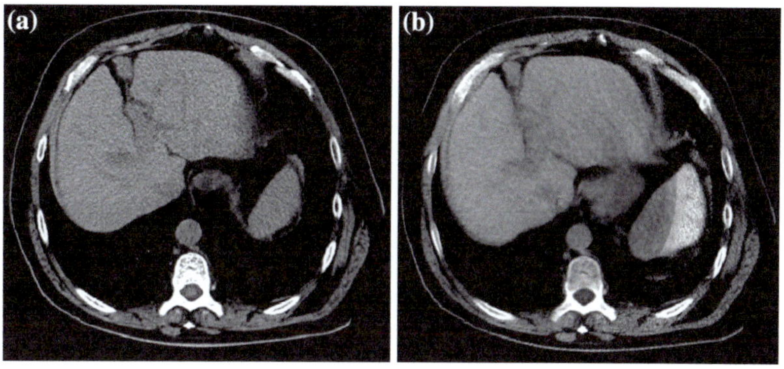

Fig. 2.3 Pre-contrast (**a**) and corresponding virtual non-contrast image (**b**) of the liver

Material differentiation, considered as the ability to distinguish different materials, including iodine [1] may be exploited in different ways.

It has been extensively investigated in vascular imaging, in which a DECT protocol in the high- and low-energy spectra has been proven useful in aortic and visceral imaging, distal runoffs, and cervical CT angiography [9].

In aortic imaging, iodine-selective maps may highlight differences between high-attenuating blood, high-attenuating bone, and iodine increasing diagnostic confidence in the evaluation of subtle endoleaks [27]. Also the ability of generating post-processed bone-subtracted three-dimensional aortic CTA images has been proven useful in clarifying complex vascular anatomy and related abnormalities [28].

In peripheral CTA, bone subtraction using a DECT approach has been shown to be a superior and faster option against conventional bone segmentation [29, 30]; unfortunately, incomplete subtraction and vascular truncation may occur [31]. Despite that, in comparison to DSA, a dual-energy bone-subtracted peripheral CTA is highly sensitive, specific, and accurate (94–97 %) [32]. Calcific plaque removal may also be an advantageous application, although has been observed to better perform in the aorto-iliac tract rather than distal segments [33]. It has been demonstrated that also highly calcified plaques may be removed from vessel walls at post-processing both in phantom [34] and in vivo [35] studies.

In the evaluation of intracranial vessels, DECT angiography with bone subtraction appears to be more accurate and faster than threshold-based bone subtraction. Residual bone and vessel truncation is usually present with the threshold-based method, due to narrow space between enhancing vessels and bony structure [36]. In comparison to mask-subtracted CTA, DECT proved to deliver similar diagnostic results [37]. Calcified plaque removal and characterization using DECT has been also demonstrated in the intracranial vascular evaluation with promising results [38–41].

Relatively to *contrast material differentiation and quantification* is acknowledged that iodine attenuation increases approximately by a two-fold factor at 80 kVp compared with 140 kVp. Therefore, an increase in iodine conspicuity may be observed at lower-kVp imaging both in dual-energy studies and low-kVp mono-energetic acquisitions [23]. This concept has been applied both to hypervascular [22] and hypovascular lesions [42] in the liver, considering for the latter the advantage of a higher lesion-background contrast difference.

The ability of selectively discriminating iodine allows its subtraction and the eventual display of its distribution. Therefore, virtual non-contrast imaging is another feasible clinical application of DECT that allows selective iodine subtraction [43, 44] and also dose reduction [45].

Virtual non-contrast imaging is an algorithm-based subtraction technique [46]. Virtual images have been proven an acceptable substitute of standard non-enhanced pre-contrast imaging [44], with a dose decrease up to 50 % [47]. Clinical application and usefulness has been demonstrated both in abdominal [7] and vascular imaging [9] (Fig. 2.3).

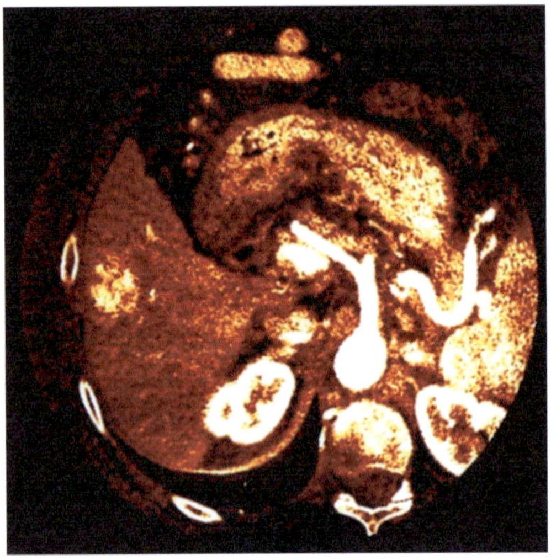

Fig. 2.4 Color-coded Iodine distribution map derived from a DECT study of the liver. Note the *right lobe* hypervascular liver lesion along with the exquisite overall vascular depiction

Iodine color-coded imaging and iodine perfusion maps follow the same principle and allow quantitative display of iodine concentration (Fig. 2.4). These applications have been proven useful in genitourinary [47–49], thoracic [50, 51], and cardiovascular [52, 53] imaging.

In aortic imaging, advantages of dual-spectra acquisitions may be applied to improve poorly opacified studies and enhance visualization of small vascular branches. The lower energy acquisition may aid in recognition of subtle endoleaks in the perigraft space after repair [20, 54, 55]. In general, we suggest evaluating both energy acquisitions along with blended images in order to enhance diagnostic accuracy, during DECT studies reading (Fig. 2.5).

It has been demonstrated that endoleak attenuation is higher at lower energies [55]. A single DECT-delayed acquisition has been proposed as a possible approach in post-treatment EVAR evaluation, with the advantage of dose reduction [56, 57].

In aortic CT angiography, the standard CT protocol includes unenhanced images to detect intramural hematoma or vessel calcifications especially in dissections and performance of virtual non-contrast imaging from a DECT protocol has been consequently evaluated. In this setting, it has been confirmed that a virtual unenhanced reconstruction may substitute standard unenhanced images and reduce the delivered dose [58].

2.4 Spectral Imaging and Iodine

Spectral CT is presently under investigation and only limited to research environments. It relies on photon-counting detector systems and the spectral information may be used to distinguish different materials based on their K-edge [53, 59, 60]. The identification of different K-edges allows the distinction of multiple high atomic numbers elements simultaneously, allowing multi-element K-edge imaging. Iodine ($Z = 53$; K-edge = 33.2 keV) is among those elements. Unfortunately, photon starvation is a serious

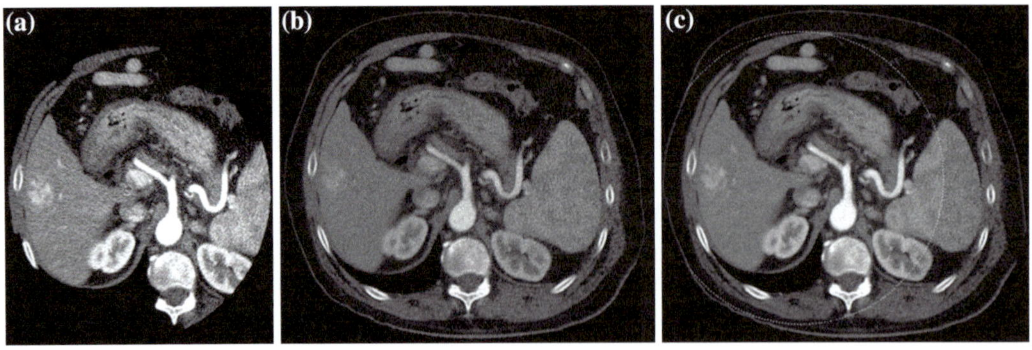

Fig. 2.5 Different iodine conspicuities demonstrated at 80 kVp (**a**) and 140 kVp (**b**) in a DECT liver study. A blended image (0.3 factor) is also presented (**c**). Note the augmented conspicuity of iodine in the lower-energy acquisition (**a**)

problem in the lower-energy range; therefore, gadolinium ($Z = 64$; K-edge = 50.2 keV) appears to be a more promising detectable agent [60]. A preliminary study has been conducted in mice where the authors demonstrated simultaneous depiction of iodine, calcium, and barium [12].

Recent introduction of the Gemstone Spectral Imaging (GSI) system (GE, Milwaukee, USA) with broad keV manipulation appears also promising in terms of material differentiation (iodine-calcium-water) and iodine mapping [61].

2.5 Low-kVp Protocols and Iodine: Conspicuity and Dose Reduction

Based on the aforementioned CT physics principles, a mono-energetic low-kVp CT acquisition, near to the iodine K-edge (K-edge = 33.2 keV), is an advantageous "contrast-enhancing" strategy. Unfortunately, a mono-energetic low-kVp CT acquisition has the drawback of a higher noise and a high-tube-current setting is necessary to decrease it [23]. Clinical applications of mono-energetic low kVp have been described in vascular [28, 62, 63], abdominal [23, 64], and neck [25] contrast-enhanced CT protocols demonstrating both contrast-enhanced conspicuity and dose lowering.

In particular, Schindera et al. performed an in vitro experimental study evaluating depiction of simulated hypervascular lesions along with noise, contrast-to-noise ratio, lesion conspicuity, and dose for a low-voltage high-current CT protocol [65]. Their experiment included CT analysis of different concentration of iodinated solutions (from 4.0 to 5.4 mg I/mL) scanned at 140, 120, 100, and 80 kVp with an indirectly proportional mAs increment. Results of their study demonstrated 45 % of noise increase using an 80-kVp protocol compared to 140-kVp. Despite the noise increase, the lower-energy protocol had the highest contrast-to-noise ratio, the highest contrast conspicuity and the lowest delivered radiation dose, demonstrating potential advantages of eventually adopting such imaging strategy.

Recently, CT manufacturers are introducing iterative reconstruction (IR) techniques (ASIR, MBIR, IRIS, AIDR, iDose) to compensate for image noise when using lower tube voltage settings. A dose decreases up to 65 %, when using a low-kVp iteratively reconstructed abdominal CT protocol has been observed [23, 66–69].

Interestingly Cho and colleagues compared two different mono-energetic CT protocols at different energies (80 vs. 120 kVp) using two different iodinated contrast concentrations (300 vs. 370 mg/mL) for CT angiography of the renal arteries [63]. Results of their study indicated that using an 80-kVp protocol with moderately concentrated contrast media (300 mg/mL) might improve arterial enhancement delivering high image quality, using a smaller amount of iodine and lower radiation dose. The authors advocate the use of this imaging strategy to potentially reduce the risk of contrast-induced nephropathy in high-risk patients.

2.6 Conclusion

In conclusion, dual- and multi-energy computed tomographs are able to differentiate materials based on tissue analysis relatively to energy and matter interaction. To better understand the rationale behind material differentiation, thus iodinated contrast media behavior in multi-energy CT studies, the relation between tube kilovoltage and K-edge for iodine should always be recalled.

Latest generation tomographs are able to deliver a broad energy spectrum (kVp) and high power (mAs). Powerful hardware combined with novel software algorithms allows fascinating post-processing techniques such as selective subtraction imaging (virtual imaging) and iodine distribution mapping among others.

Dual-energy imaging is currently available in most advanced diagnostic centers while spectral imaging is still in an early and experimental phase.

Radiologists and clinicians should be familiar with DECT technical features and iodine-energy-related characteristics to exploit this novel technique in the clinical setting.

Mono-energetic low-kVp CT protocols may be also used to exploit iodine behavior in the lower-energy spectra.

References

1. Johnson TR, Krauss B, Sedlmair M, Grasruck M, Bruder H, Morhard D et al (2007) Material differentiation by dual energy CT: initial experience. Eur Radiol 17(6):1510–1517
2. Coursey CA, Nelson RC, Boll DT, Paulson EK, Ho LM, Neville AM et al (2010) Dual-energy multidetector CT: how does it work, what can it tell us, and when can we use it in abdominopelvic imaging? Radiographics 30(4):1037–1055
3. Fornaro J, Leschka S, Hibbeln D, Butler A, Anderson N, Pache G et al (2011) Dual- and multi-energy CT: approach to functional imaging. Insights Imaging 2(2):149–159
4. Bauer RW, Kramer S, Renker M, Schell B, Larson MC, Beeres M et al (2011) Dose and image quality at CT pulmonary angiography-comparison of first and second generation dual-energy CT and 64-slice CT. Eur Radiol 21(10):2139–2147
5. Kalender WA, Perman WH, Vetter JR, Klotz E (1986) Evaluation of a prototype dual-energy computed tomographic apparatus. I. Phantom Stud. Med Phys. 13(3):334–339
6. Kalender WA (2005) CT: the unexpected evolution of an imaging modality. Eur Radiol 15(Suppl 4):D21–D24
7. Silva AC, Morse BG, Hara AK, Paden RG, Hongo N, Pavlicek W (2011) Dual-energy (spectral) CT: applications in abdominal imaging. Radiographics, 31(4): 1031–1046; discussion 47–50
8. Remy-Jardin M, Faivre JB, Pontana F, Hachulla AL, Tacelli N, Santangelo T et al (2010) Thoracic applications of dual energy. Radiol Clin North Am 48(1):193–205
9. Vlahos I, Chung R, Nair A, Morgan R (2012) Dual-energy CT: vascular applications. AJR Am J Roentgenol 199(5 Suppl):S87–S97
10. Desai MA, Peterson JJ, Garner HW, Kransdorf MJ (2011) Clinical utility of dual-energy CT for evaluation of tophaceous gout. Radiographics, 31(5): 1365–1375; discussion 76–7
11. Gupta R, Phan CM, Leidecker C, Brady TJ, Hirsch JA, Nogueira RG et al (2010) Evaluation of dual-energy CT for differentiating intracerebral hemorrhage from iodinated contrast material staining. Radiology 257(1):205–211
12. Anderson NG, Butler AP, Scott NJ, Cook NJ, Butzer JS, Schleich N et al (2010) Spectroscopic (multi-energy) CT distinguishes iodine and barium contrast material in MICE. Eur Radiol 20(9):2126–2134
13. Rutherford RA, Pullan BR, Isherwood I (1976) X-ray energies for effective atomic number determination. Neuroradiology 11(1):23–28
14. Millner MR, McDavid WD, Waggener RG, Dennis MJ, Payne WH, Sank VJ (1979) Extraction of information from CT scans at different energies. Med Phys 6(1):70–71
15. Compton AH (1923) A quantum theory of the scattering of X-rays by light Elements. Phys Rev 21(5):483–502
16. Bushberg JT (1998) The AAPM/RSNA physics tutorial for residents. X-ray interactions. Radiographics 18(2):457–468
17. Riederer SJ, Mistretta CA (1977) Selective iodine imaging using K-edge energies in computerized x-ray tomography. Med Phys 4(6):474–481
18. Abudurexiti A, Kameda M, Sato E, Abderyim P, Enomoto T, Watanabe M et al (2010) Demonstration of iodine K-edge imaging by use of an energy-discrimination X-ray computed tomography system with a cadmium telluride detector. Radiol Phys Technol 3(2):127–135
19. Wintersperger B, Jakobs T, Herzog P, Schaller S, Nikolaou K, Suess C et al (2005) Aorto-iliac multidetector-row CT angiography with low kV settings: improved vessel enhancement and simultaneous reduction of radiation dose. Eur Radiol 15(2):334–341
20. Schueller-Weidekamm C, Schaefer-Prokop CM, Weber M, Herold CJ, Prokop M (2006) CT angiography of pulmonary arteries to detect pulmonary embolism: improvement of vascular enhancement with low kilovoltage settings. Radiology 241(3):899–907
21. Yeh BM, Shepherd JA, Wang ZJ, Teh HS, Hartman RP, Prevrhal S (2009) Dual-energy and low-kVp CT in the abdomen. AJR Am J Roentgenol 193(1):47–54
22. Marin D, Nelson RC, Samei E, Paulson EK, Ho LM, Boll DT et al (2009) Hypervascular liver tumors: low tube voltage, high tube current multidetector CT during late hepatic arterial phase for detection–initial clinical experience. Radiology 251(3):771–779
23. Marin D, Nelson RC, Schindera ST, Richard S, Youngblood RS, Yoshizumi TT et al (2010) Low-tube-voltage, high-tube-current multidetector abdominal CT: improved image quality and decreased radiation dose with adaptive statistical iterative reconstruction algorithm–initial clinical experience. Radiology 254(1):145–153
24. Yeh BM, Abdominal CT (2011) At low peak tube potential settings brings promises, but new rules apply. AJR Am J Roentgenol 196(6):1322–1323
25. Gnannt R, Winklehner A, Goetti R, Schmidt B, Kollias S, Alkadhi H (2012) Low kilovoltage CT of the neck with 70 kVp: comparison with a standard protocol. AJNR Am J Neuroradiol 33(6):1014–1019

26. McNitt-Gray MF (2002) AAPM/RSNA physics tutorial for residents: topics in CT radiation dose in CT. Radiographics 22(6):1541–1553
27. Ascenti G, Mazziotti S, Lamberto S, Bottari A, Caloggero S, Racchiusa S et al (2011) Dual-energy CT for detection of endoleaks after endovascular abdominal aneurysm repair: usefulness of colored iodine overlay. AJR Am J Roentgenol 196(6): 1408–1414
28. Godoy MC, Naidich DP, Marchiori E, Leidecker C, Schmidt B, Assadourian B et al (2010) Single-acquisition dual-energy multidetector computed tomography: analysis of vascular enhancement and postprocessing techniques for evaluating the thoracic aorta. J Comput Assist Tomogr 34(5):670–677
29. Sommer WH, Johnson TR, Becker CR, Arnoldi E, Kramer H, Reiser MF et al (2009) The value of dual-energy bone removal in maximum intensity projections of lower extremity computed tomography angiography. Invest Radiol 44(5): 285–292
30. Yamamoto S, McWilliams J, Arellano C, Marfori W, Cheng W, McNamara T et al (2009) Dual-energy CT angiography of pelvic and lower extremity arteries: dual-energy bone subtraction versus manual bone subtraction. Clin Radiol 64(11):1088–1096
31. Meyer BC, Werncke T, Hopfenmuller W, Raatschen HJ, Wolf KJ, Albrecht T (2008) Dual energy CT of peripheral arteries: effect of automatic bone and plaque removal on image quality and grading of stenoses. Eur J Radiol 68(3):414–422
32. Brockmann C, Jochum S, Sadick M, Huck K, Ziegler P, Fink C et al (2009) Dual-energy CT angiography in peripheral arterial occlusive disease. Cardiovasc Intervent Radiol 32(4):630–637
33. Thomas C, Korn A, Ketelsen D, Danz S, Tsifikas I, Claussen CD et al (2010) Automatic lumen segmentation in calcified plaques: dual-energy CT versus standard reconstructions in comparison with digital subtraction angiography. AJR Am J Roentgenol 194(6):1590–1595
34. Werncke T, Albrecht T, Wolf KJ, Meyer BC (2010) Dual energy CT of the peripheral arteries: a phantom study to assess the effect of automatic plaque removal on stenosis grading. Rofo. 182(8):682–689
35. Uotani K, Watanabe Y, Higashi M, Nakazawa T, Kono AK, Hori Y et al (2009) Dual-energy CT head bone and hard plaque removal for quantification of calcified carotid stenosis: utility and comparison with digital subtraction angiography. Eur Radiol 19(8): 2060–2065
36. Morhard D, Fink C, Graser A, Reiser MF, Becker C, Johnson TR (2009) Cervical and cranial computed tomographic angiography with automated bone removal: dual energy computed tomography versus standard computed tomography. Invest Radiol 44(5):293–297
37. Lell MM, Kramer M, Klotz E, Villablanca P, Ruehm SG (2009) Carotid computed tomography angiography with automated bone suppression: a comparative study between dual energy and bone subtraction techniques. Invest Radiol 44(6):322–328
38. Ma R, Liu C, Deng K, Song SJ, Wang DP, Huang L (2010) Cerebral artery evaluation of dual energy CT angiography with dual source CT. Chin Med J (Engl). 123(9):1139–1144
39. Henzler T, Porubsky S, Kayed H, Harder N, Krissak UR, Meyer M et al (2011) Attenuation-based characterization of coronary atherosclerotic plaque: comparison of dual source and dual energy CT with single-source CT and histopathology. Eur J Radiol 80(1):54–59
40. Watanabe Y, Nakazawa T, Higashi M, Itoh T, Naito H (2011) Assessment of calcified carotid plaque volume: comparison of contrast-enhanced dual-energy CT angiography and native single-energy CT. AJR Am J Roentgenol 196(6):W796–W799
41. Postma AA, Hofman PA, Stadler AA, van Oostenbrugge RJ, Tijssen MP, Wildberger JE (2012) Dual-energy CT of the brain and intracranial vessels. AJR Am J Roentgenol 199(5 Suppl):S26–S33
42. Robinson E, Babb J, Chandarana H, Macari M (2010) Dual source dual energy MDCT: comparison of 80 kVp and weighted average 120 kVp data for conspicuity of hypo-vascular liver metastases. Invest Radiol 45(7):413–418
43. Zhang LJ, Peng J, Wu SY, Wang ZJ, Wu XS, Zhou CS et al (2010) Liver virtual non-enhanced CT with dual-source, dual-energy CT: a preliminary study. Eur Radiol 20(9):2257–2264
44. Toepker M, Moritz T, Krauss B, Weber M, Euller G, Mang T et al (2012) Virtual non-contrast in second-generation, dual-energy computed tomography: reliability of attenuation values. Eur J Radiol 81(3):e398–e405
45. Yu L, Liu X, Leng S, Kofler JM, Ramirez-Giraldo JC, Qu M et al (2009) Radiation dose reduction in computed tomography: techniques and future perspective. Imaging Med 1(1):65–84
46. Petersilka M, Bruder H, Krauss B, Stierstorfer K, Flohr TG (2008) Technical principles of dual source CT. Eur J Radiol 68(3):362–368
47. Graser A, Becker CR, Staehler M, Clevert DA, Macari M, Arndt N et al (2010) Single-phase dual-energy CT allows for characterization of renal masses as benign or malignant. Invest Radiol 45(7):399–405
48. Gupta RT, Ho LM, Marin D, Boll DT, Barnhart HX, Nelson RC (2010) Dual-energy CT for characterization of adrenal nodules: initial experience. AJR Am J Roentgenol 194(6): 1479–1483
49. Leschka S, Stolzmann P, Baumuller S, Scheffel H, Desbiolles L, Schmid B et al (2010) Performance of dual-energy CT with tin filter technology for the discrimination of renal cysts and enhancing masses. Acad Radiol 17(4):526–534
50. Pansini V, Remy-Jardin M, Faivre JB, Schmidt B, Dejardin-Bothelo A, Perez T et al (2009) Assessment

of lobar perfusion in smokers according to the presence and severity of emphysema: preliminary experience with dual-energy CT angiography. Eur Radiol 19(12):2834–2843

51. Thieme SF, Johnson TR, Lee C, McWilliams J, Becker CR, Reiser MF et al (2009) Dual-energy CT for the assessment of contrast material distribution in the pulmonary parenchyma. AJR Am J Roentgenol 193(1):144–149
52. Ruzsics B, Lee H, Zwerner PL, Gebregziabher M, Costello P, Schoepf UJ (2008) Dual-energy CT of the heart for diagnosing coronary artery stenosis and myocardial ischemia-initial experience. Eur Radiol 18(11):2414–2424
53. Schwarz F, Ruzsics B, Schoepf UJ, Bastarrika G, Chiaramida SA, Abro JA et al (2008) Dual-energy CT of the heart–principles and protocols. Eur J Radiol 68(3):423–433
54. Gorgos A, Remy-Jardin M, Duhamel A, Faivre JB, Tacelli N, Delannoy V et al (2009) Evaluation of peripheral pulmonary arteries at 80 kV and at 140 kV: dual-energy computed tomography assessment in 51 patients. J Comput Assist Tomogr 33(6):981–986
55. Szucs-Farkas Z, Semadeni M, Bensler S, Patak MA, von Allmen G, Vock P et al (2009) Endoleak detection with CT angiography in an abdominal aortic aneurysm phantom: effect of tube energy, simulated patient size, and physical properties of endoleaks. Radiology 251(2):590–598
56. Chandarana H, Godoy MC, Vlahos I, Graser A, Babb J, Leidecker C et al (2008) Abdominal aorta: evaluation with dual-source dual-energy multidetector CT after endovascular repair of aneurysms–initial observations. Radiology 249(2):692–700
57. Stolzmann P, Frauenfelder T, Pfammatter T, Peter N, Scheffel H, Lachat M et al (2008) Endoleaks after endovascular abdominal aortic aneurysm repair: detection with dual-energy dual-source CT. Radiology 249(2):682–691
58. Numburi UD, Schoenhagen P, Flamm SD, Greenberg RK, Primak AN, Saba OI et al (2010) Feasibility of dual-energy CT in the arterial phase: imaging after endovascular aortic repair. AJR Am J Roentgenol 195(2):486–493
59. Roessl E, Proksa R (2007) K-edge imaging in x-ray computed tomography using multi-bin photon counting detectors. Phys Med Biol 52(15): 4679–4696
60. Schlomka JP, Roessl E, Dorscheid R, Dill S, Martens G, Istel T et al (2008) Experimental feasibility of multi-energy photon-counting K-edge imaging in pre-clinical computed tomography. Phys Med Biol 53(15):4031–4047
61. Zhang D, Li X, Liu B (2011) Objective characterization of GE discovery CT750 HD scanner: gemstone spectral imaging mode. Med Phys 38(3):1178–1188
62. Fujikawa A, Matsuoka S, Kuramochi K, Yoshikawa T, Yagihashi O, Kurihara Y et al (2011) Vascular enhancement and image quality of CT venography: comparison of standard and low kilovoltage settings. AJR Am J Roentgenol 197(4):838–843
63. Cho ES, Yu JS, Ahn JH, Kim JH, Chung JJ, Lee HK et al (2012) CT angiography of the renal arteries: comparison of lower-tube-voltage CTA with moderate-concentration iodinated contrast material and conventional CTA. AJR Am J Roentgenol 199(1):96–102
64. Marin D, Nelson RC, Barnhart H, Schindera ST, Ho LM, Jaffe TA et al (2010) Detection of pancreatic tumors, image quality, and radiation dose during the pancreatic parenchymal phase: effect of a low-tube-voltage, high-tube-current CT technique–preliminary results. Radiology 256(2):450–459
65. Schindera ST, Nelson RC, Mukundan S Jr, Paulson EK, Jaffe TA, Miller CM et al (2008) Hypervascular liver tumors: low tube voltage, high tube current multi-detector row CT for enhanced detection–phantom study. Radiology 246(1):125–132
66. Hara AK, Paden RG, Silva AC, Kujak JL, Lawder HJ, Pavlicek W (2009) Iterative reconstruction technique for reducing body radiation dose at CT: feasibility study. AJR Am J Roentgenol 193(3):764–771
67. Schindera ST, Diedrichsen L, Muller HC, Rusch O, Marin D, Schmidt B et al (2011) Iterative reconstruction algorithm for abdominal multidetector CT at different tube voltages: assessment of diagnostic accuracy, image quality, and radiation dose in a phantom study. Radiology 260(2):454–462
68. Martinsen AC, Saether HK, Hol PK, Olsen DR, Skaane P (2012) Iterative reconstruction reduces abdominal CT dose. Eur J Radiol 81(7):1483–1487
69. Mitsumori LM, Shuman WP, Busey JM, Kolokythas O, Koprowicz KM (2012) Adaptive statistical iterative reconstruction versus filtered back projection in the same patient: 64 channel liver CT image quality and patient radiation dose. Eur Radiol 22(1):138–143

3 Renal Masses

Giorgio Ascenti, Achille Mileto, Bernhard Krauss,
Silvio Mazziotti, Carmelo Sofia and Emanuele Scribano

3.1 Introduction

Renal masses are commonly detected during imaging of the kidneys. It has been estimated that over half of patients over the age of 50 years harbor at least one renal mass, most commonly a simple cyst. In particular, most of renal masses are discovered incidentally when an imaging examination is performed to evaluate a non-renal complaint. Although most represent benign renal cysts, not all incidental renal masses are benign, and most renal cell carcinoma (RCC) are also incidentally discovered in this scenario. Therefore, differentiating incidental benign renal masses from those that are potentially malignant is the most important challenge in daily practice [1–5].

RCC is the eight most common malignancy and according to estimates by the American Cancer Society, it was newly diagnosed in 64,000 people in the United States in 2012, and approximately 14,000 are expected to die of the disease [6].

The 2004 World Health Organization classification is now adopted and worldwide accepted for classification of renal tumors (Table 1). This classification distinguishes six types of renal tumors, based on histologic matrix arising (renal cell; metanephric; mixed mesenchymal and epithelial; nephroblastic, neuroendocrine; other origins). In particular, among renal cell tumors, benign and malignant are distinguished. Moreover, this classification lists inherited or familial predisposition (known inherited syndromes) to renal neoplasms, which is present in less than 4 % of renal tumors [7].

Clear cell-type RCC is the most frequent variant, accounting to 80 % of all cases of renal tumors. Most clear cell RCC are solitary cortical neoplasms that occur with equal frequency in either kidney; multicentricity (4 %) and bilaterality (0.5–3.0 %) may be seen. Clear cell-type RCC has a worse prognosis compared with other histologic subtypes [8].

Papillary carcinoma, which accounts to 10 % of all renal cell carcinomas, has a less aggressive clinical course than RCC clear cell type. Papillary carcinoma has variable proportions of papillae and may be bilateral or multifocal with frequent hemorrhage, necrosis, and cystic degeneration. Cellular type 1 and type 2 tumors have been recognized with papillae covered by small cells with scanty cytoplasm arranged in a single layer in type 1, and tumor cells of higher nuclear grade, eosinophilic cytoplasm and pseudostratified nuclei in type 2 [7–9].

Multilocular cystic-type RCC is considered a specific entity in the current WHO classification [7], with an incidence ranging between 1 and 4 % of all renal tumors. Multilocular cystic RCC has excellent outcome and appears entirely composed of cysts of variable size, which are lined by a single layer of clear cells small papillae, and are separated from the kidney by a fibrous capsule.

Chromophobe-type RCC is less aggressive than other RCC types and accounts for 5 % of renal epithelial tumors. Some authors suggest a

G. Ascenti et al., *CT of the Retroperitoneum*,
DOI: 10.1007/978-88-470-5469-1_3, © Springer-Verlag Italia 2014

Table 1 WHO classification of renal tumors (modified from Ref. [7])

Familial renal cancer
Renal cell tumors
Malignant
Clear cell renal cell carcinoma
Multilocular clear cell renal cell carcinoma
Papillary renal cell carcinoma
Chromophobe renal cell carcinoma
Carcinoma of the collecting ducts of Bellini
Renal medullary carcinoma
Xp11 translocation carcinomas
Carcinoma associated with neuroblastoma
Mucinous tubular and spindle cell carcinoma
Renal cell carcinoma unclassified
Benign
Papillary adenoma
Oncocytoma
Metanephric tumors
Metanephric adenoma
Metanephric adenofibroma
Metanephric stromal tumors
Mixed mesenchymal and epithelial tumors
Cystic nephroma
Mixed epithelial and stromal tumor
Synovial sarcoma
Nephroblastic tumors
Nephrogenic rests
Nephroblastoma
Cystic partially differentiated nephroblastoma
Neuroendocrine tumors
Carcinoid
Neuroendocrine carcinoma
Primitive neuroectodermal tumor
Neuroblastoma
Phaeochromocytoma
Other tumors
Mesenchymal tumors
Hematopoietic and lymphoid tumors
Germ cell tumors
Metastatic tumors

relationship between chromophobe-type RCC and oncocytoma, with the foregoing which is thought to be the benign counterpart of chromophobe-type RCC [10]. Collecting duct and medullary-type RCC carcinoma accounts up to 2 % of all cases of renal tumors. While the collecting duct type derives from the “principal cells” of the collecting duct, medullary-type RCC is a rapidly growing rare tumor of the renal medulla. Several authors regard the medullary-type as an aggressive variant of the collecting duct-type RCC [11].

Oncocytoma and angiomyolipoma are the two most common benign lesions of the kidney.

Oncocytoma comprises 3–9 % of all primary renal neoplasms. Males are affected twice as often as females. Due to the absence of peculiar macroscopic imaging findings, lesions are challenging to distinguish from RCC. Renal angiomyolipomas (AML) are hamartomas composed of vascular, smooth muscle, and mature fat. The majority of angiomyolipomas are sporadic (80 %) and are typically identified in adults; the remaining 20 % are syndromic. They can usually have characteristic imaging appearances [9–12].

Besides these types of renal masses, common daily findings are benign renal cysts. The overwhelming majority of renal cysts are found by chance in the general population and are detected on US or CT in more than 50 % of patients older than 50 years [13]. Most renal cysts represent benign “leave alone” renal cortical lesions and require neither surgical resection nor follow-up imaging. Uncommonly, however, RCC can present as a complex cystic renal lesion and thus, it is mandatory to distinguish benign cysts from cystic RCC [14].

RCC, as in general most of renal masses, may remain clinically occult for most of its course. The classic triad of flank pain, hematuria, and flank mass is uncommon (10 %), and it is indicative of advanced disease in patients with RCC. Twenty-five to thirty percent of patients are asymptomatic, and their RCC are found on incidental uroradiologic or abdominal imaging study [15].

3.2 State of the Art of Conventional (Multidetector) CT

MDCT is the mainstay in the characterization and staging of renal masses. When one is specifically asked to characterize a renal mass with CT, the examination needs to be performed before and after administration of intravenous contrast material [5, 13, 16].

Pre-contrast images are used for baseline density measurements in both solid and complex cystic masses but also provide information about morphological and structural features, such as the presence of intralesional fat or calcium.

Post-contrast images are used to evaluate enhancement, defined as delta of CT density measured on pre- and post-contrast images. Although contrast-enhancement do not necessarily indicate malignancy of a renal mass, either solid (i.e., oncocytoma and angiomyolipoma with no macroscopic fat) either complex cystic (i.e., inflammatory cyst), it represents the diagnostic clue that permits to differentiate surgery-needing from non-surgery-needing renal masses.

After intravenous contrast material administration, three different phases of renal enhancement are acquired: the corticomedullary phase, in which there is corticomedullary differentiation and which occurs 20–70 s after the injection of contrast material; the nephrographic phase, in which there is a homogeneous maximally enhanced nephrogram and which occurs 80–120 s after the injection of contrast material; the excretory phase, in which the nephrogram is homogeneous, but there is decreased enhancement of the parenchyma because contrast material has been excreted into the collecting system and which occurs 5-10 min after the administration of contrast material (Fig. 3.1) [17, 18].

The nephrographic phase is ideal to detect and characterize renal masses. Because there is maximal and homogeneous parenchymal enhancement, this allows better detection of renal masses, which typically do not enhance to the same degree as the renal parenchyma. The corticomedullary and excretory phases occasionally may make the detection of renal masses more difficult. During the corticomedullary phase, small renal masses may be indistinguishable from the renal medulla; during the excretory phase, renal masses may be of the same attenuation as the renal parenchyma, which has de-enhanced [17, 18].

During the nephrographic phase, most of renal neoplasms are maximally enhanced. Because the identification of enhancement is necessary to diagnose a neoplasm, maximal enhancement of neoplasms is especially important in the hypovascular ones (papillary RCC). In these cases, the unequivocal demonstration of enhancement is challenging because papillary renal cell carcinomas are particularly prone to enhance less and at a slower rate than other tumors [19]. Imaging in the corticomedullary phase is useful in showing the normal corticomedullary pattern in pseudotumors such as prominent columns of Bertin, as in depicting renal vasculature for a nephron-sparing surgery [20]. Furthermore, the typical hypervascular pattern of clear cell renal carcinoma can be demonstrated in this phase. Imaging in the excretory phases is required when an involvement of the excretory system is suspected [16–19].

When encountering any renal mass, it is necessary to first determine whether the detected abnormality represents a pseudotumor, a mass-like finding that mimics a neoplasm. Renal pseudotumors are caused by a variety of conditions including congenital anomalies (prominent renal column of Bertin, dromedary humps) (Fig. 3.2), inflammatory masses (focal pyelonephritis, chronic renal abscess, and autoimmune disease), vascular structures (renal artery aneurysm or arteriovenous fistula), or abnormalities relating to trauma or hemorrhage. Although some renal pseudotumors require treatment, they are treated differently from neoplasms, and therefore, their recognition is important to ensure proper management. If they are not first excluded when evaluating a renal mass-like finding, the application of image-based criteria used to evaluate renal masses could lead to an incorrect diagnosis. For example, enhancement

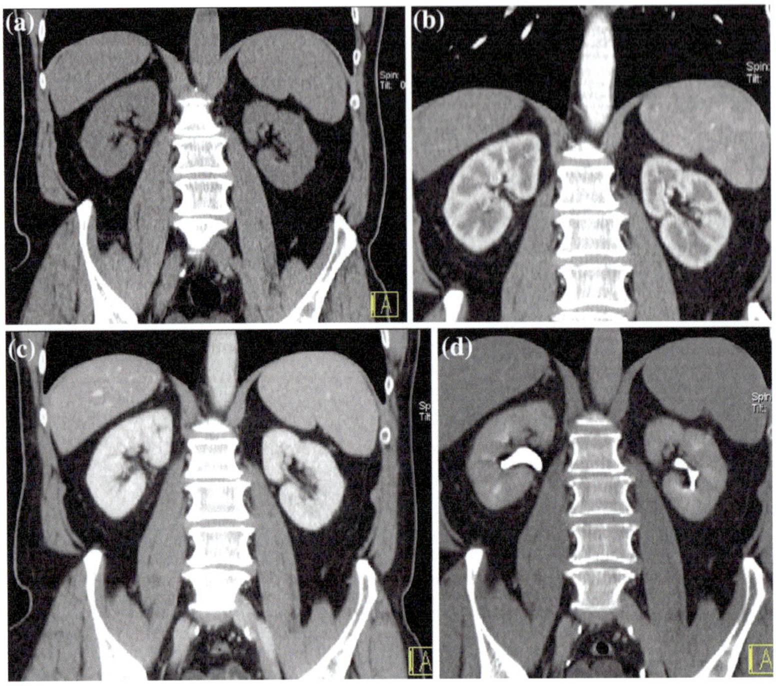

Fig. 3.1 Example of different MDCT renal protocol study phases. Coronally reformatted unenhanced (**a**), corticomedullary (**b**), nephrographic (**c**), and excretory (**d**) phases

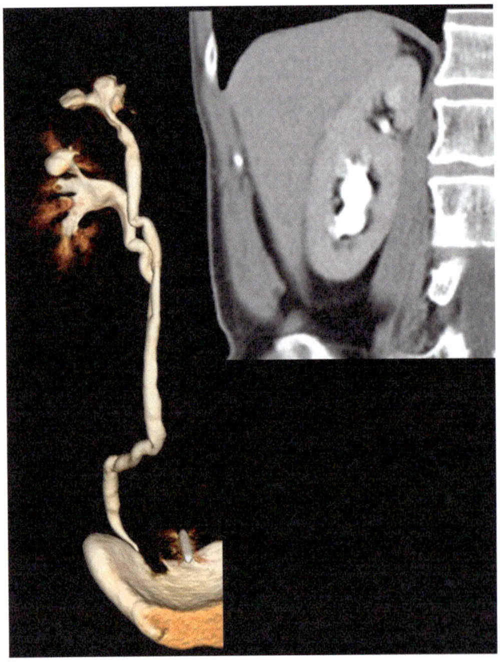

Fig. 3.2 Volume-rendering and coronally reformatted nephrographic phase images in a patient with hypertrophic Bertin column associated with double collecting system

is often used to support the diagnosis of a neoplasm, but enhancement can be found in infectious and other inflammatory conditions, aneurysms, and vascular malformations. Key radiologic features to support an inflammatory cause include ill-defined margins and perinephric fat stranding. Aneurysms and vascular malformations enhance similar to nearby vasculature; in the case of a vascular malformation, hypertrophy of the ipsilateral renal artery and arteriovenous shunting may be present. Finally, in the presence of a renal pseudotumor, the same degree of enhancement respect to normal parenchyma in all study phases is the diagnostic clue [20].

Once pseudotumors are excluded, mass enhancement indicates a neoplasm (Fig. 3.3). Renal mass enhancement is affected by multiple factors: the amount and rate of the contrast material injected, scan delay, and the vascularity of the mass. Highly vascular tumors show marked enhancement, whereas hypovascular tumors show minimal enhancement. There is no universally agreed upon specific value that can

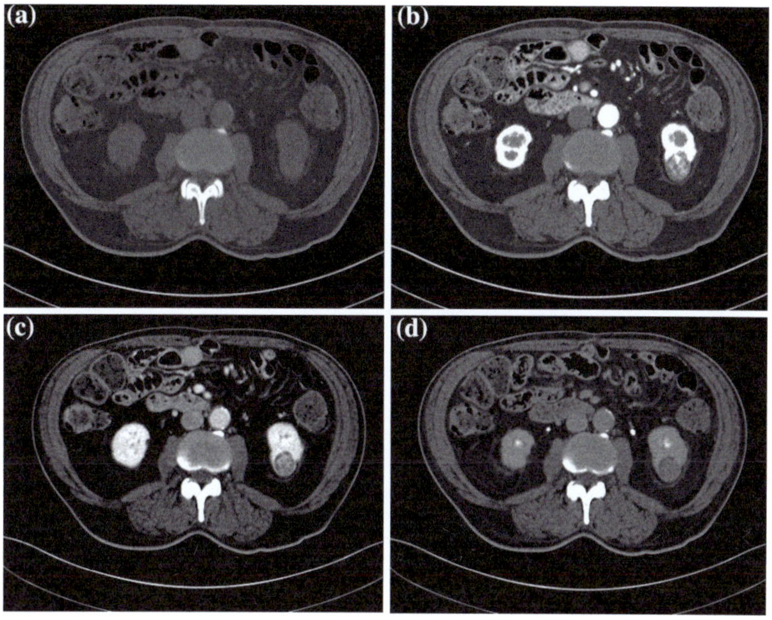

Fig. 3.3 Unenhanced (**a**) and contrast-enhanced corticomedullary (**b**), nephrographic (**c**), excretory (**d**) study phases in a patient with RCC, clear cell type, of the left kidney

be used as a cutoff point for differentiating non-enhancing cysts from enhancing solid tumors. In MDCT, a threshold of 20 HU is worldwide used to indicate definitive enhancement within a renal mass, values of 10–19 HU as equivocal for enhancement, and values of less than 10 HU as indicating no enhancement [5, 20].

Cystic lesions are the most commonly detected renal masses, with most being benign simple cysts. Simple cysts are defined as having a hairline-thin wall, no septa or calcification, and being filled with simple fluid that measures 0–20 HU (Fig. 3.4). There are no soft-tissue components within simple cysts; they do not enhance after the administration of contrast medium, and they are considered benign [21–23]. When a cystic renal mass contains material showing attenuation higher than simple fluid (>20 HU), one or more septa, calcifications, thickened walls or septa, or enhancing soft-tissue components, it cannot be considered a simple cyst. The Bosniak classification system has been used worldwide in evaluating cystic renal masses over the past 25 years. Cystic renal masses are classified into 5 groups based on CT findings: categories I, II, IIF, III, and IV [22, 24–26]. Category I masses are simple cysts and are always benign. Category II masses are minimally complicated cysts that can be reliably considered as benign. They may contain a few (generally 1 or 2) hairline-thin septa in which perceived (not measurable) enhancement may be appreciated. The wall or septa may contain fine calcifications or a short segment of slightly thickened smooth calcification. High-attenuation cysts $\leq$3 cm are also included in category II (Fig. 3.5). These masses were initially described as containing attenuation higher than renal parenchyma (typically 40–90 HU), but the attenuation criterion has been expanded to include masses with attenuations more than 20 HU. To diagnose a high-attenuation cyst, the mass must be well circumscribed, homogeneously high-attenuating and must not enhance. Homogeneity is an important feature; high-attenuation fluid within a renal mass may mask small regions of enhancement. Therefore, it is important to obtain multiple attenuation measurements of varying sizes throughout the lesion to ensure that the mass is homogeneous and that no portion of the mass enhances [20, 22, 25, 27].

Category IIF lesions are likely benign but require follow-up imaging to show stability. These masses may contain multiple hairline-thin

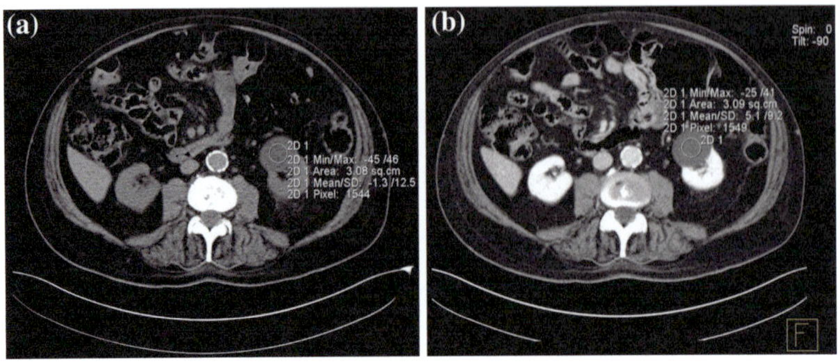

Fig. 3.4 Axial unenhanced (**a**) and contrast-enhanced nephrographic (**b**) phase images in a patient with left renal simple cyst. The lesion shows baseline water density (**a**) and no contrast-enhancement on nephrographic phase image is seen (**b**)

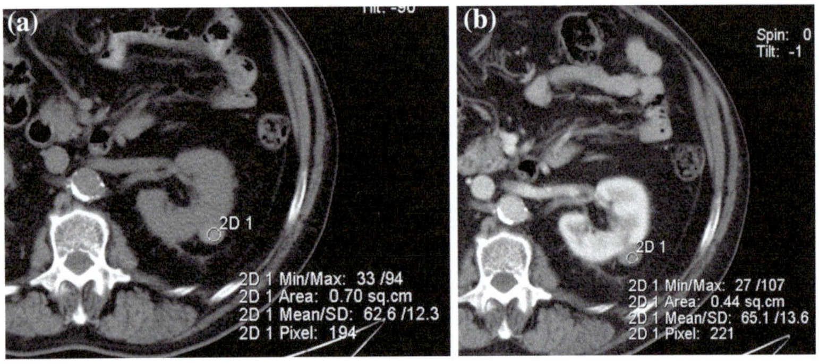

Fig. 3.5 Axial unenhanced (**a**) and contrast-enhanced nephrographic (**b**) phase images in a patient with high-attenuation (Bosniak category II) cyst of the left kidney. The lesion shows baseline high-density (**a**), consistent with hemorrhagic content, and no contrast-enhancement on nephrographic phase image is seen (**b**)

septa in which enhancement may be visually perceived (not measurable enhancement). Category IIF renal masses may contain thick or nodular calcification, with no soft tissue enhancing nodules. Non-enhancing high-attenuation renal cysts that measure more than 3 cm are included. Category IIF masses should be followed for morphologic and structural changes, such as development of septa, wall thickening, or new areas of enhancement, suggestive of malignancy. Growth is not a useful determinant of malignancy, because simple benign cysts may grow and renal cell carcinomas may not. Therefore, growth is not a feature of the Bosniak renal cyst classification [22–27]. The recommended interval for follow-up examinations is to obtain a CT scan or MR imaging examination at 6 and 12 months, followed by yearly examinations for a minimum of 5 years. However, there is no known time interval of stability that can be used to diagnose a renal mass as benign with complete certainty. However, whether a Bosniak category IIF lesion has not significantly morphologically changed in a period of 5 years, it is likely benign [22].

Category III cysts are truly indeterminate masses because they have a reasonable probability of being benign or malignant. Imaging features include a thickened wall or septa that show measurable enhancement. Benign masses in this category include acute and chronically infected cysts, hemorrhagic cysts (often secondary to trauma), benign multiseptated cysts, and cystic neoplasms such as multilocular cystic nephroma. Malignant masses in this category include multilocular cystic RCC. Initially, it was

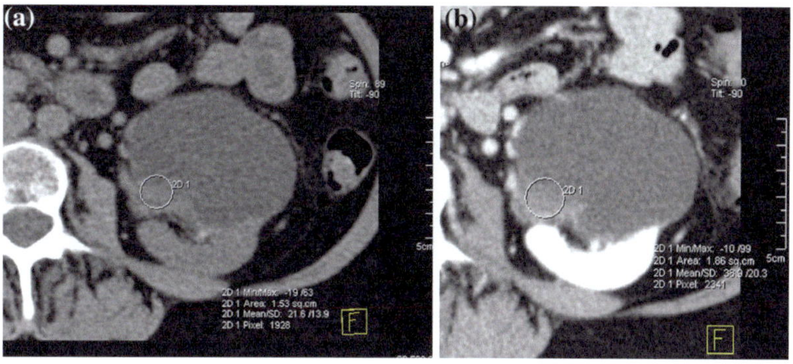

Fig. 3.6 Axial unenhanced (**a**) and contrast-enhanced nephrographic phase (**b**) images in a patient with cystic RCC (Bosniak category IV). The lesion shows a mural nodule with soft-tissue baseline density (**a**) that has moderate enhancement on nephrographic phase image (**b**)

estimated that approximately half of category III masses were benign and the other half were malignant. Recent studies have shown a wide range (31–100 %) of these masses to be malignant. This wide variation may be attributed either to radiologists' experience in renal mass imaging or to practice of referring urologists caring for the patient. Since category IIF was introduced, most category III renal masses that were previously removed are now being followed (category IIF), with a subsequent greater percentage of malignant category III masses remaining. Surgery remains the preferred treatment if the patient does not have high surgical risk [5, 22, 25].

Finally, category IV cysts are clearly malignant masses until proved otherwise and therefore require surgical removal. Imaging features include those described in category III with the additional presence of nodular enhancement within the mass or adjacent to its wall (Fig. 3.6). The probability of such a mass being malignant is close to 100 % [22–30].

Although there are well-established, time-tested, image-based criteria, it is often very difficult distinguishing benign complicated from malignant cystic renal masses mainly due to the overlap between the gross morphologic and radiologic findings. Thus, characterization of complex cystic renal masses , as malignant lesions requiring surgery and non-malignant lesions that do not, remains a common diagnostic challenge [28–30].

A solid renal mass is best defined as having little or no fluid components and usually consists predominantly of enhancing soft-tissue. As detailed earlier, after excluding pseudotumors, a solid renal mass should be considered a renal neoplasm. In particular, whether a solid renal mass enhances by more than 20 HU, or whether it shows enhancement in the simultaneous presence of calcification and macroscopic fat, it has to be considered as RCC until proven otherwise and pathology is mandatory (Fig. 3.7) [5, 17, 20]. It is also necessary to diagnose those malignant renal neoplasms that do not require surgery (e.g., lymphoma and metastatic disease). A combination of clinical history and imaging findings may allow these masses to be diagnosed. However, in some cases, percutaneous biopsy may be required. When there is a history of an extra-renal primary tumor, the 50–85 % of solitary renal masses are metastatic. Therefore, if a solid renal mass is detected in a patient with a known primary malignancy (e.g., lung cancer, lymphoma), a metastasis should not be necessarily diagnosed presumptively; both a second primary (RCC) and a benign neoplasm should be considered [5, 17, 20].

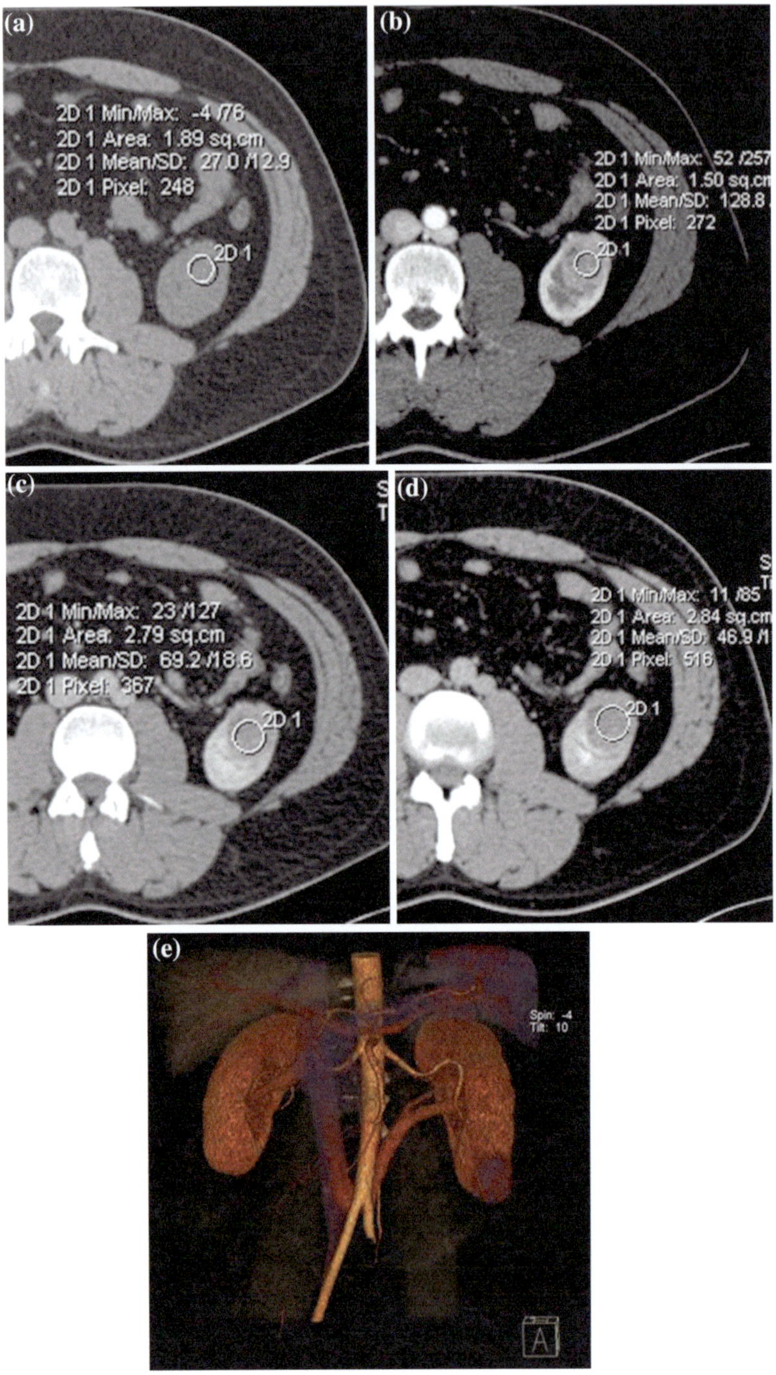

Fig. 3.7 Axial unenhanced (**a**), contrast-enhanced corticomedullary (**b**), nephrographic (**c**) and excretory (**d**) study phases, with corresponding VR image (**e**) in a patient with RCC, clear cell type, of the left kidney. The lesion shows soft-tissue baseline density (**a**) and enhancement after contrast-medium administration (**b**, **c**). This nodule has moderate enhancement on nephrographic phase image (**c**) and progressively de-enhances on excretory phase image (**d**)

However, many small (≤3 cm) solid renal masses are benign [31]. Benign diagnoses typically encountered at surgery, for what was previously believed to be RCC mainly include oncocytomas and angiomyolipomas.

Oncocytoma is a benign solid renal mass that cannot be differentiated from RCC by imaging. Although a central scar or homogeneous enhancement at CT or MRI is suggestive of oncocytoma, these findings are not specific and a tissue diagnosis is necessary to differentiate oncocytoma from RCC [31–33].

Angiomyolipoma is a benign neoplasm that, particularly when small, warrants no treatment. Most angiomyolipomas can be diagnosed by identifying regions of fat within a non-calcified renal mass at unenhanced CT. Some angiomyolipomas contain very small quantities of fat that can be overlooked if the mass is not carefully evaluated. However, approximately 5 % of angiomyolipomas do not contain fat that can be seen at imaging, and the differentiation from other renal neoplasms is not possible with CT. These masses, referred to as angiomyolipoma with minimal fat, are often small, mildly hyperattenuating on unenhanced CT examination and homogeneously enhanced with contrast material. However, these findings are not specific enough to make a confident diagnosis of an angiomyolipoma, and other tumors, such as papillary RCC, metanephric adenoma, oncocytoma and leiomyoma, may have a similar appearance [34, 35].

Further problems in enhancement evaluation, mainly due to multiphasic acquisition, i.e., different positioning of region-of-interest (ROI) on sequential images or difficulty with appropriate placement of a ROI in intrarenal tumors that are isodense to parenchyma on unenhanced image, make sometimes a definitive diagnosis difficult at MDCT, especially when small hypovascular tumors are encountered. Another frequent problem is represented by the pseudoenhancement, which is defined as an artificial elevation of the HU attenuation of a simple renal cyst imaged on contrast-enhanced CT image during nephrographic phase, at peak of parenchymal enhancement. Pseudoenhancement is thought to be principally due to the image reconstruction algorithms used to adjust for beam-hardening artifacts [36, 37].

3.3 Spectral CT: Study Protocols and Clinical Applications

By means of spectral analysis, dual-energy imaging provide complementary information and approach toward a new hybrid, morphologic-functional imaging.

Various clinically relevant applications have been established for dual-energy CT renal lesion imaging [38–45]. These applications can be distinguished in *non-material-specific*, *material-specific,* and *energy-specific* (Fig. 3.8).

Non-material-specific applications permit to enhance the iodine image conspicuity while optimizing the contrast-to-noise ratio. The two datasets obtained from dual-energy acquisition at high and low kVp can be separately analyzed or blended in a single image stack. In particular, high-energy images have the advantage of lowered noise scan, but at the same time, this advantage is offset by the decrease in contrast resolution. On the other hand, low-energy images show a better contrast resolution, but the acquired dataset is nosier (Fig. 3.8) [39–41].

Both to exploit benefits and to alleviate drawbacks of both kVp scans fused (140- and 80-kVp) datasets with an intermediate weighting and different blending strategies have been developed. The first used approach was a linear-blending fashion that uses a simple linear-blending algorithm using fixed percentages of 80- and 140-kVp datasets. Several studies, both in vitro and in vivo, demonstrated that a linear-blending ratio of 70 % 140-kVp and 30 % 80-kVp have image characteristics similar to a standard single-energy scan and thus can be considered a simulated weighted-average 120-kVp dataset (Fig. 3.8). On second-generation dual-source scanner, the linear-blending ratio of 50 % from 100-kVp and 50 % from 140-kVp datasets has image characteristics similar to a standard 120-kVp single-energy scan. However, the application of a fixed weighting factor for all pixels reduces both noise and high contrast [46–48]. The second strategy, alternative to linear blending, is represented by non-linear image-blending mode (Fig. 3.8). The goal of this mixing strategy is to maintain the contrast of the low-energy scan, while achieving the noise characteristics of the high-energy scan. In particular, the high-intensity regions corresponding to iodine contrast-enhancement are preferentially extracted by 80-kVp data, to maintain the high image contrast in regions of high iodine concentration. By contrast, low-intensity levels, which correspond to air, water, and soft tissues,

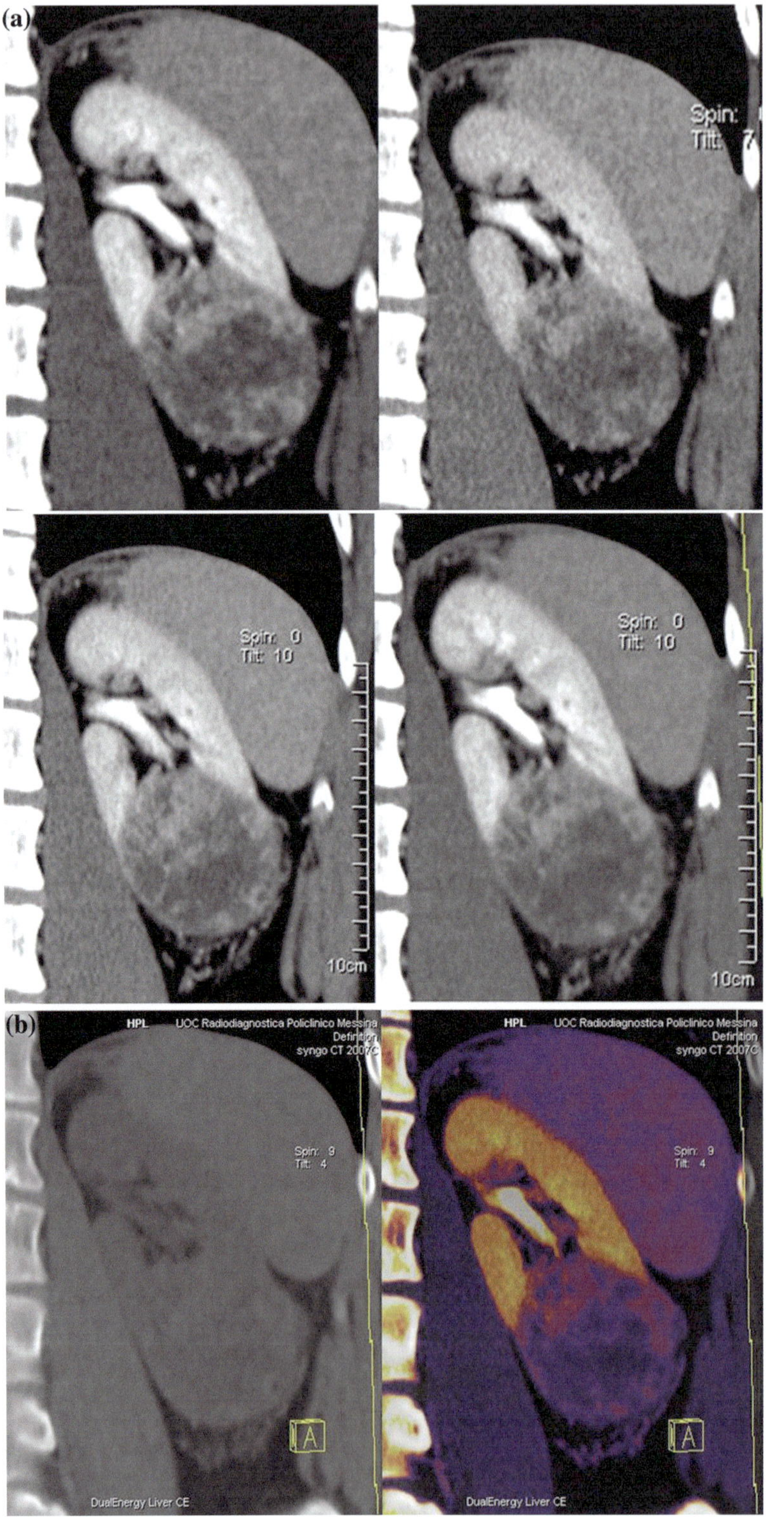

Fig. 3.8 Dual-energy *non-material-specific* (**a**), *material-specific* (**b**) and *energy-specific* (**c**) applications in a patient with RCC, clear cell type, of the left kidney. The low-kVp (*upper left corner*) and high-kVp (*upper right corner*) can be separately analyzed (**a**) or blended in a single image stack in either a linear (*lower left corner*) or alternatively in a non-linear fashion (*lower right corner*). Based on a three-material decomposition algorithm (**b**) iodine spectral extraction image series is created, with virtual unenhanced (*left*) and color-coded iodine overlay image (*right*) series. By applying a mathematic computerized model to the polychromatic source data obtained from the dual-energy acquisition, separate monochromatic image series (**c**) are created

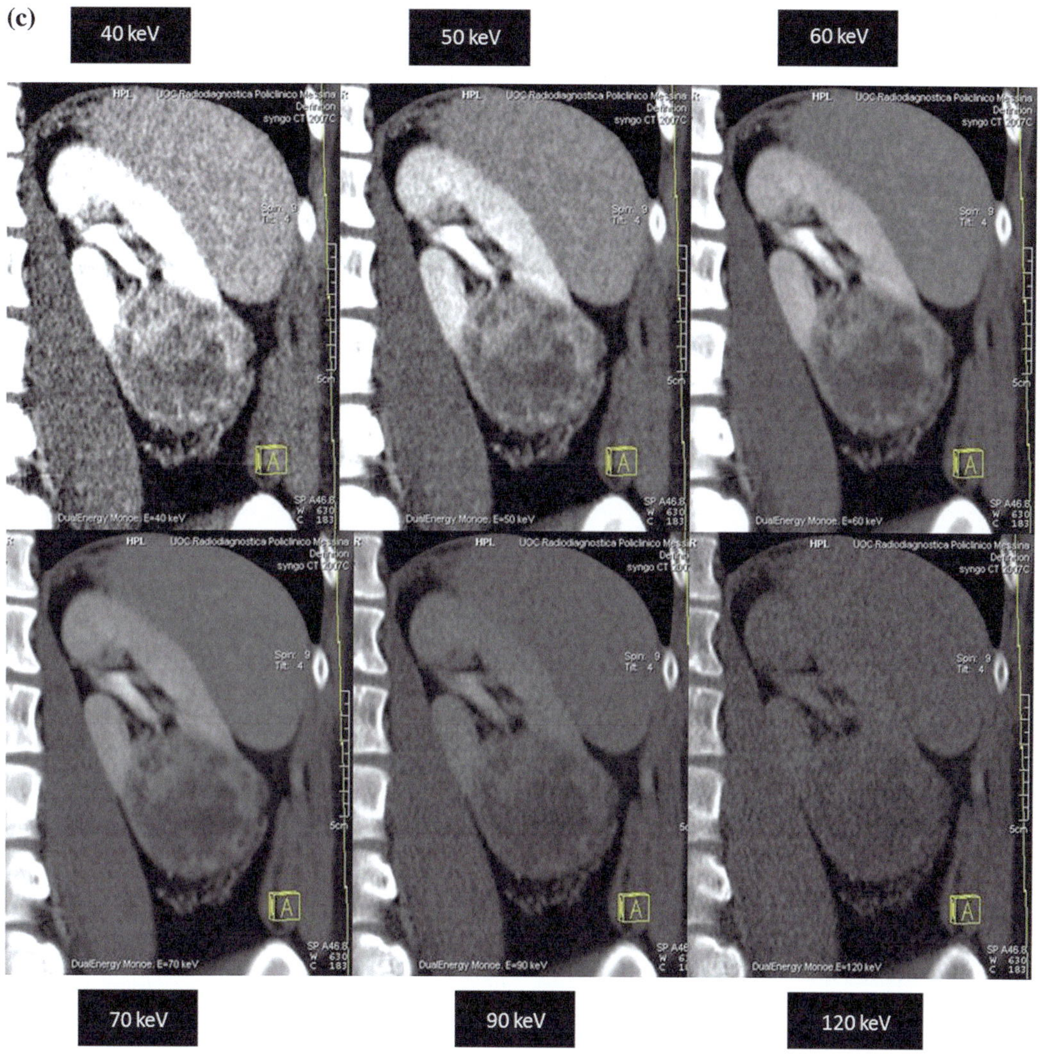

Fig. 3.8 (continued)

are less noisy in 140-kV scan and should be preferred in the blending process [49, 50]. The result is an image in which iodine signal is magnified, while optimizing contrast differences and minimizing image noise. Several non-linear-blending functions including a binary-blending function, a slope blending function, a Gaussian function, and a modified sigmoid function have been developed. Recently, a piecewise linear-blending function method has been commercially implemented in the dual-source platform (labeled as "Optimum Contrast"). A recent study has demonstrated that, compared with a standard linear-blending reconstruction algorithm, a piecewise linear-blending function method leads to significantly improve tumor conspicuity and enable better image quality in the evaluation of renal masses at DECT during nephrographic phase of enhancement [51]. This can be useful in defining neoplastic or inflammatory renal medullary pyramids infiltration and permits to reduce the flow rate and amount of administered contrast medium in patients with mild impairment of renal function.

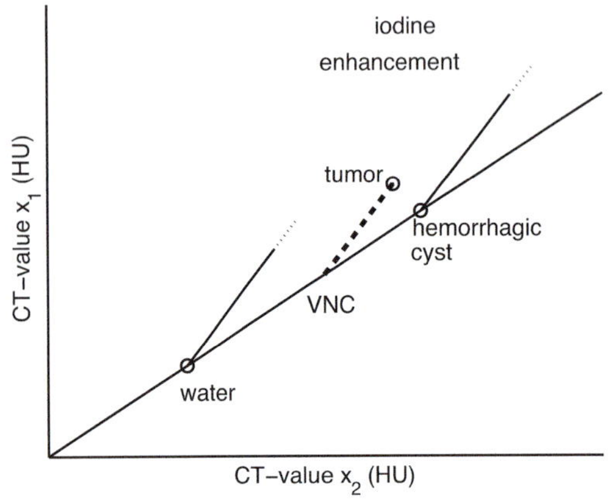

Fig. 3.9 Drawing shows how material decomposition into iodine and water is used to calculate the iodine enhancement and virtual non-contrast images. Note that there is a simple parallel projection in the CT-value diagram

Material-specific applications, mainly based on three- or two-material-decomposition principles, allow the reader to differentiate, isolate and quantitate different materials having different *k*-edge values. This capability to extract materials improves as they show high atomic number (i.e., iodine or calcium) [39, 52, 53].

These applications are based on the fact that iodine enhancement is much higher at low tube voltage than at high tube voltage (typically a factor of 2 between 80 kV and 140 kV), whereas body soft tissues (with the exception of fat) have approximately the same CT values for both spectra. Therefore, in terms of X-ray absorption, they can be considered as being equivalent to water of a higher density. In Fig. 3.9, it is shown how material decomposition into iodine and water can be used to calculate the iodine enhancement and virtual non-contrast images based on a simple parallel projection in the CT-value diagram (Fig. 3.9).

With a dual-energy post-processing algorithm, based on the three-material decomposition principle, iodine can be subtracted or overlaid on conventional gray-scale information, and therefore, a iodine spectral-extraction series, consisting of virtual unenhanced and color-coded iodine overlay images, is achieved (Fig. 3.8) [39–41]. If the technology and scanning techniques are optimized, the necessity for a baseline-unenhanced CT acquisition could be eliminated, leading to significant reductions in radiation dose to patients.

The evaluation of cystic and solid renal masses represents one of most investigated applications of dual-energy CT technology [43, 44, 51, 52, 54, 55]. Similar to current single-energy CT imaging evaluation of a mass, the virtual-unenhanced images can be used to replace the true unenhanced CT acquisition. The attenuation of the lesion on the virtual-unenhanced series can serve as a baseline to compare with the contrast-enhanced series. Several studies [53, 54, 56] demonstrated that no significant difference in the attenuation of renal lesions between true and virtual unenhanced images exists (Fig. 3.10).

The possibility of omitting the true unenhanced scan permits to achieve a considerable radiation dose saving in renal lesions imaging [52, 53, 57].

Compared with a standard triple phase single-energy MDCT protocol, Graser et al. [53] found a 35 % radiation dose decrease if a dual-energy dual-phase protocol, with subsequent reconstruction of virtual unenhanced images, is carried out. The same author showed that it is possible to dramatically cut the patient radiation exposure up to 50 % whether a single-phase MDCT protocol is performed [52]. The radiation dose saving achievable with the use of virtual unenhanced images represents a considerable advantage in patients with complex cystic renal lesions because many of these patients need follow-up for many years. A recent study demonstrated that, in the specific clinical setting of complex cystic renal masses, dual-energy CT permits to achieve a mean dose reduction of 29 % while being able to show all possible attenuation features present in renal cyst, including liquid low-attenuation (due to liquid or necrosis), intermediate-attenuation (due to soft-tissue solid nodule or debris), high-attenuation (due to hemorrhage or protein-rich content) and calcification (Fig. 3.10) [54].

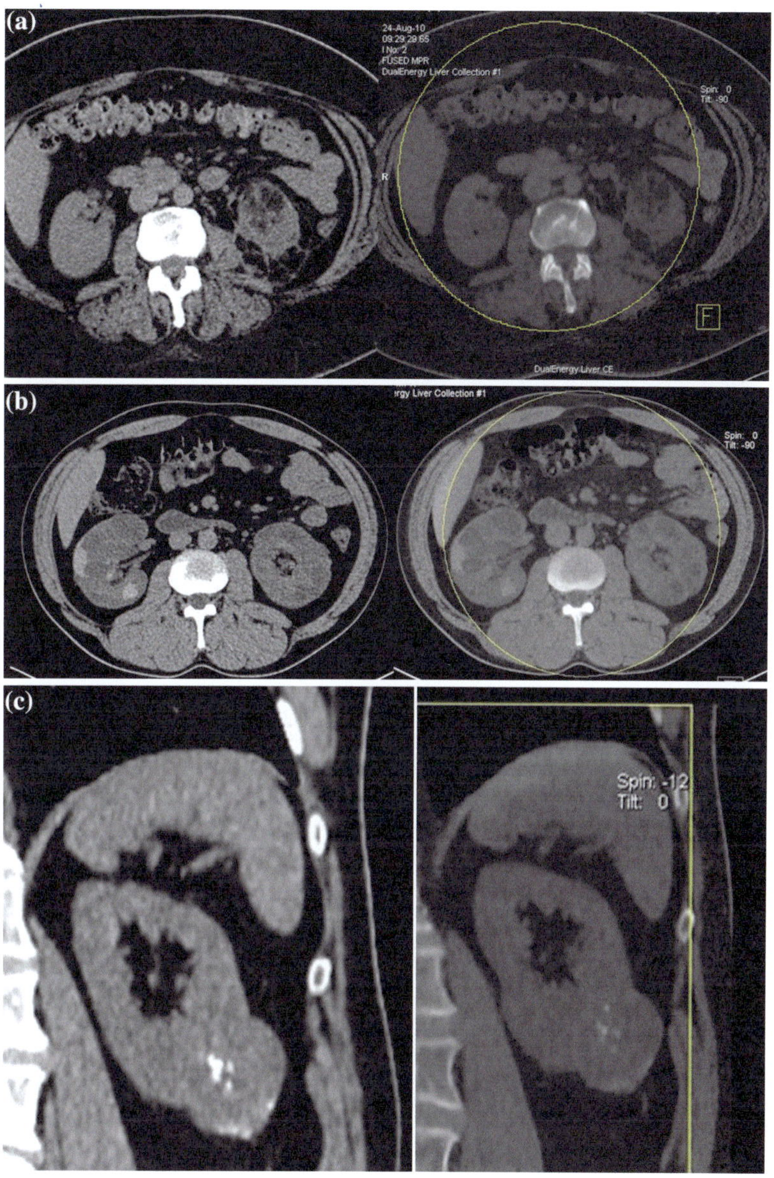

Fig. 3.10 Examples of virtual unenhanced with corresponding true unenhanced image series in lipid-rich angiomyolipoma of the left kidney (**a**), perinephric right hematoma due to hemorrhagic cyst bleeding (**b**), and solid RCC of the left kidney showing huge calcification (**c**). Note that the two image series can be easily discriminated, since virtual unenhanced images appear slightly grainier than conventional unenhanced series due to the lower kVp and smoothing induced by the post-processing algorithm. Note also the yellow ring which corresponds to the field-of-view on the tube with the smaller detector (26 cm)

Dual-energy color-coded iodine overlay images permit to immediately depict the presence of contrast medium within a mass by means of a color display. With this method, one can immediately perceive visual enhancement in a mass not relying on measured changes in attenuation (Figs. 3.11, 3.12). The direct visualization of iodine signal within the mass differentiates a cyst from a solid lesion. As renal cysts do not contain blood vessels centrally, color-coded iodine overlay image shows a cyst as devoid of iodine signal. In contrast, solid renal masses do have vessels within them, and these vessels and the tissue of the mass accumulate iodine after contrast injection. Brown first described this possible use of dual-energy CT in phantom studies, founding color-coded iodine overlay technique highly sensitive in identification of enhancing renal masses [44]. The clinical use of iodine-specific images has since been reported as well [52, 54, 57–59]. Furthermore, as found by Graser, use of a color-coded iodine overlay reduces

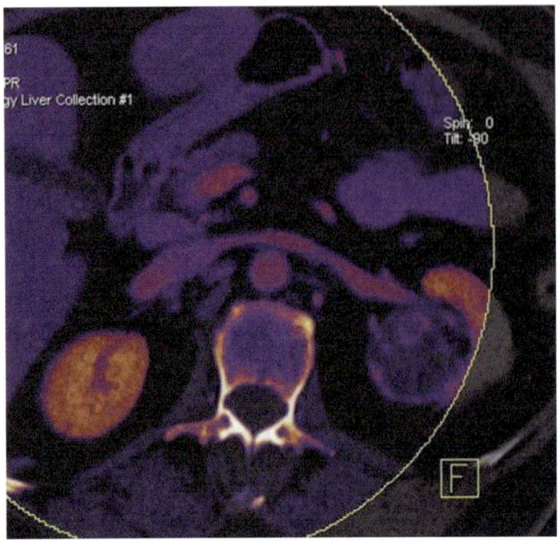

Fig. 3.11 Axial color-coded iodine overlay image in a patient with multilocular cystic left RCC. Note that the solid enhancing nodules within the tumor show iodine uptake displayed as color-coded signal, whereas the cystic areas are displayed as signal void

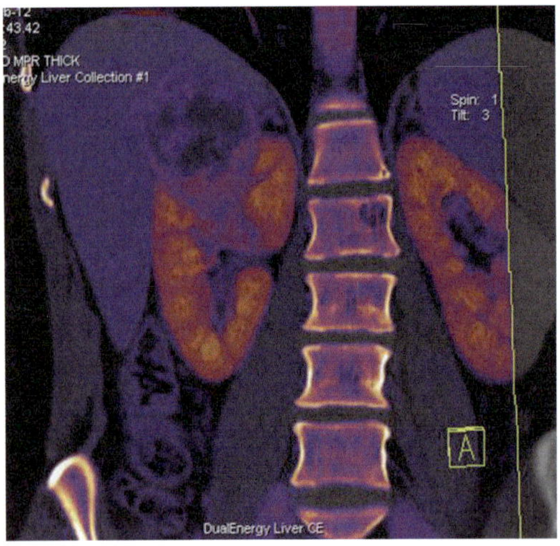

Fig. 3.12 Coronally reformatted color-coded iodine overlay image in a patient with right kidney RCC. Note that the healthy enhancing renal parenchyma as well as solid enhancing nodules within the tumor shows iodine uptake displayed as color-coded signal. Note that necrotic areas are displayed as signal void

post-processing time because enhancement can be directly quantified with the overlay function available in the dual-source dual-energy CT system, eliminating the need for double-ROI measurements and calculation of attenuation change on two images [53]. Therefore, this technique permits to overcome some problems related to multiphasic acquisition. However, this technique does not permit to address the problem of equivocal enhancement, especially in demonstrating low-level true enhancement in solid enhancing lesions (Fig. 3.13).

Overall, at dual-energy CT , there are two different ways to quantify the iodine uptake of a lesion. Firstly, it is possible to measure the iodine enhancement of the lesion, similar to the comparison of unenhanced and contrast-enhanced images with single-energy CT. As an alternative approach independent of attenuation measurement, the lesion iodine concentration (in mg/mL) can be calculated. This approach provides a more direct measure of lesion vascularity (Fig. 3.14).

Chandarana [59] found that iodine quantification with dual-energy CT is accurate in a phantom model and that the presence of an iodine concentration greater than 0.5 mg/mL in a renal lesion was equivalent to the diagnosis of enhancement on basal and contrast-enhanced acquisitions. The author supposed that qualitative or quantitative depiction of iodine may be superior to attenuation measurements, especially in discriminating minimally enhancing tumors, such as papillary subtypes of renal cancer, from high-attenuation cysts [59].

Recently, Ascenti et al. [60] demonstrated that spectral-based dual-energy CT iodine quantification is more accurate than standard enhancement measurements in distinguishing enhancing from non-enhancing renal masses , especially in depicting minimally enhancing neoplasms, such as papillary RCC and/or in excluding enhancement in small renal cysts (Figs. 3.15 and 3.16).

Kaza et al. [43] using a single-source fast-kilovoltage switching dual-energy CT reported a series of 83 renal lesions. These authors found that a measured iodine density threshold of 2 mg/cm3 had the highest accuracy (92.8 %) in detecting enhancing renal masses with a sensitivity of 90 % and specificity of 93 %.

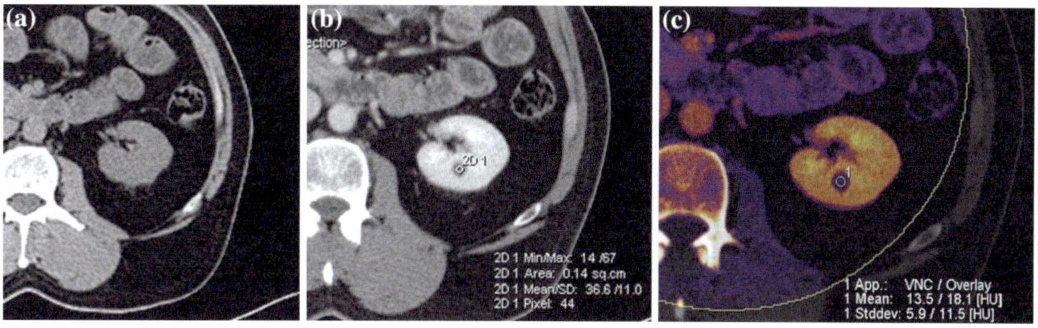

Fig. 3.13 Small left intra-renal simple cyst. **a** unenhanced single energy; **b** contrast-enhanced nephrographic phase dual-energy linear-blended (M 0.3); **c** contrast-enhanced nephrographic phase dual-energy color-coded iodine overlay. The small hypodense intrarenal lesion is visible only in nephrographic phase; (**b**) the delta of attenuation cannot be accurately evaluated in conventional imaging. Whereas dual-energy evaluation demonstrated a virtual basal attenuation of 13 HU, the enhancement of lesion remain equivocal. The attenuation increase of 18 HU is more probably due to pseudoenhancement, though a small hypovascular tumor cannot be excluded

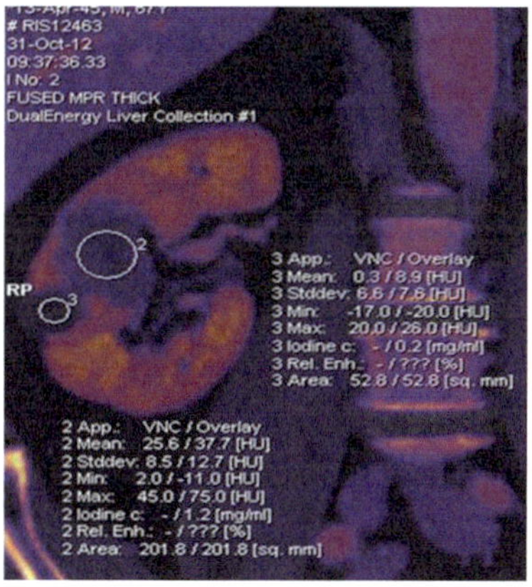

Fig. 3.14 Coronally-reformatted color-coded iodine overlay image in a patient having RCC, clear cell type, and simple cyst of the right kidney. Note that RCC shows iodine uptake, expressed by a single ROI as iodine-based enhancement (*Overlay*) and iodine concentration (in mg/mL); conversely, simple cyst does not show any iodine uptake

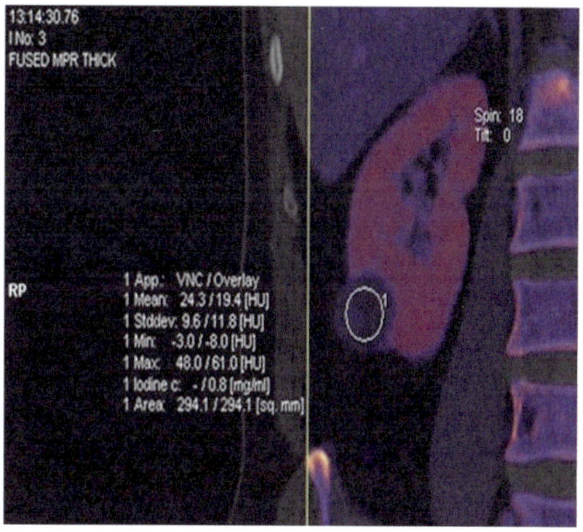

Fig. 3.15 Coronally reformatted color-coded iodine overlay image in a patient with RCC, clear cell type, of the right kidney. Note that while the lesion shows borderline attenuation-based enhancement, an evident iodine uptake is seen whether the iodine concentration is considered

Therefore, these differences in the cutoff point value reported between the two main hardware platforms need to be explained and further investigated.

More recently, Liu et al., showed that D-value (defined as the absolute difference between the CT value at 80 and 140 kVp images) and dual-energy ratio (called as CT value with 80 kV divided by the value with 140 kV) indexes are useful parameters for distinguishing homogeneously high-attenuation renal cysts from enhancing solid renal masses using a single phase dual-energy MDCT protocol. A D-value of 17.6 HU and a dual-energy ratio of 1.3 were found as most accurate cutoff point for enhancement detection [61]. Similar results were previously reported in a phantom experiment using a second-generation dual-source system [62].

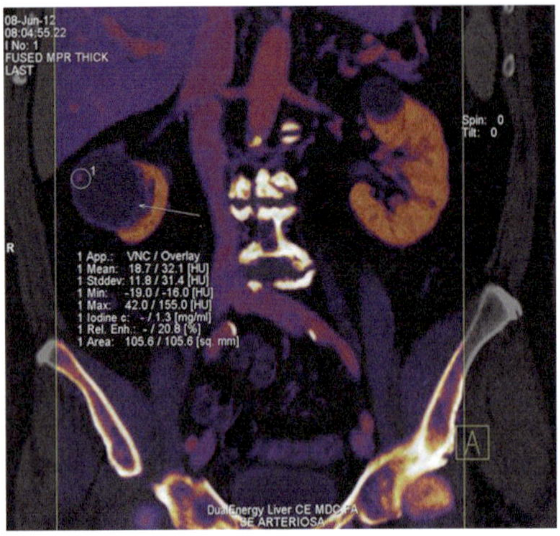

Fig. 3.16 Coronally reformatted color-coded iodine overlay image in a patient having a right kidney complex cyst and left kidney simple cyst. Note the enhancing irregular thick wall (*arrow*) and the enhancing nodule (ROI) of the neoplastic complex cyst. The absence of vascularization of the simple left cyst is seen

Finally, iodine quantification in dual-energy CT seems to have a potential to reduce renal pseudoenhancement of small simple or hyper-attenuating cysts (Figs. 3.17 and 3.18).

Based on material decomposition and the knowledge of mass attenuation of materials, dual-energy enables *energy-specific* application, represented by the creation of virtual monochromatic images. In particular, a mathematic computerized model is applied to the polychromatic source data obtained from the dual-energy acquisition. However, whether a single-source fast-kVp switching platform is used, monochromatic images are synthesized in the data domain, whereas for dual-energy CT, data acquired with dual-source CT systems, image domain basis material decomposition is typically used. This is due to the fact that projection data deriving from the low- and high-energy scans are collected by the dual-source system in helical mode, and thus, data are not coincident one with each other. For a given photon energy, virtual monochromatic images, whose energy is reported as kiloelectronvolts (keV) instead of peak voltage (kVp), mimic those images that would result from a true monochromatic X-ray source. The advantage of a monochromatic beam is that it is less susceptible to beam-hardening artifact and therefore has the potential to provide more accurate and more reproducible attenuation measurements over conventional MDCT. Preliminary experiences show that monochromatic images permit to alleviate the pseudoenhancement phenomenon in renal cysts [63]. Similar results are obtained in a phantom study using a second-generation dual-source system [64].

Furthermore, with the use of dedicated software applications, keV spectral attenuation curves can be generated by plotting the attenuation values (in HU) of a material at different monochromatic energies, ranging from 40 to 140 keV. With this technique, specific tissue characterization is achievable based on known mean attenuation characteristics of different materials, especially those with higher atomic numbers, enhancing solid renal lesions may be therefore differentiated from non-enhancing cysts in a single-phase nephrographic image on the basis of the attenuation curves (Fig. 3.19) [65, 66]. In particular, iodine-containing lesions show an upwardly steep curve at the decrease of energy levels, whereas avascular cysts show relatively flat curves at all energies; these curves can be also normalized using the healthy renal parenchyma as reference background. By indirectly identifying the iodine uptake, this method may also open new perspective to assess response to therapy and tumor viability.

Overall, the choice of study phase for the dual-energy scan is the first step, and it depends on the specific clinical scenario. If a renal mass (e.g., previously detected by US examination) has to be characterized the best CT phase for performing the dual-energy scan is the nephrographic phase. In this setting, all advantages of dual-energy CT images in the enhancement analysis can be exploited. Conversely, whether a patient with a known renal mass undergoes CT for staging, the opportunity of performing the dual-energy scan during the corticomedullary

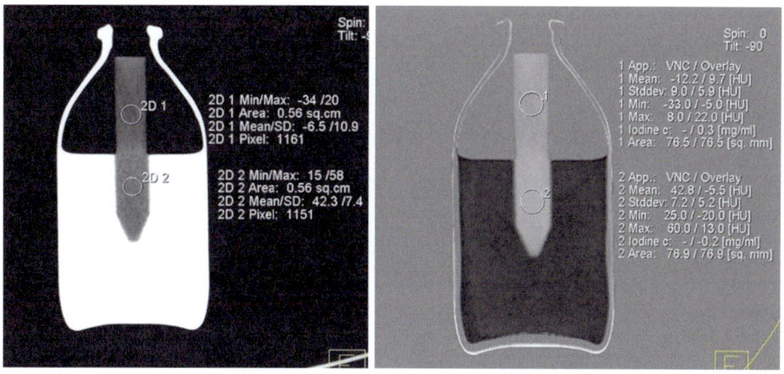

Fig. 3.17 Standard 120-kVp (*on the left*) and corresponding dual-energy color-coded iodine overlay (*on the right*) images of a phantom containing a vial of water immersed in an iodine solution (20 mg/mL). The lower ROI on the standard 120-kVp image clearly demonstrates pseudoenhancement, whereas the ROI at the corresponding level on DE image shows no surreptitious elevation of attenuation. Iodine quantification in mg/mL confirms the absence of iodine into the vial (−0.2 mg/mL)

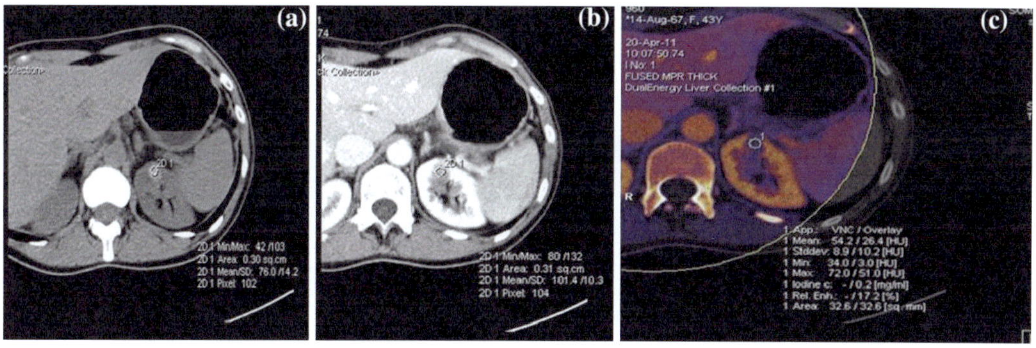

Fig. 3.18 Small hyperdense intraparenchimal left renal cyst showing pseudoenhancement at conventional CT evaluation. Axial CT images. **a** unenhanced single-energy phase; **b** contrast-enhanced nephrographic phase dual-energy linear-blended (M 0.3); **c** contrast-enhanced nephrographic phase dual energy with color-coded iodine overlay. The basal attenuation of the cyst (76 HU) increased of 25 HU mimicking enhancement of a solid lesion. In such case, a renal tumor as a papillary carcinoma cannot be excluded. Diagnosis of hyperdense cyst is confidently made for the absence of iodine into the lesion (0.2 mg/mL)

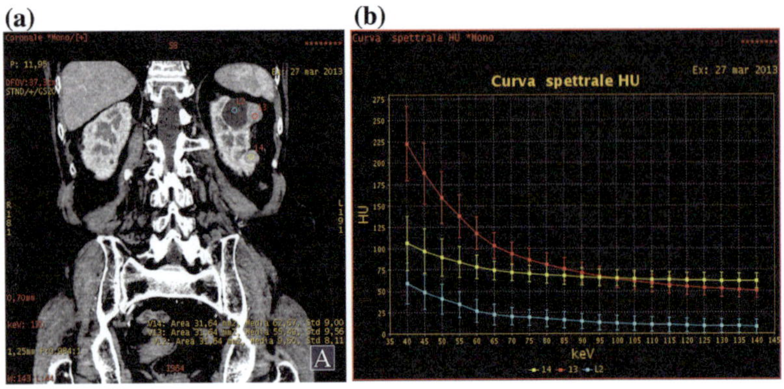

Fig. 3.19 Renal cell carcinoma, simple and high-attenuation left renal cyst. **a** Monochromatic DECT image (120 keV) shows a hypoattenuating left renal lesion (*light blue ROI*) and two hyperattenuating left renal lesions (*red and yellow ROI*). The first lesion is likely to be a cyst (attenuation < 10 HU). The remaining two lesions have an indeterminate appearance that could be represents either an enhancing mass or a high-attenuation cyst. **b** the graphic shows DECT spectral attenuation curves for the three lesions at various kiloelectron-volt values. The hypodense (*light blue ROI*) and one high-attenuation (*yellow ROI*) lesions have flat curves, indicating that they are avascular. The first is a simple cyst and the latter is a hemorrhagic or a proteinaceous cyst. The remaining hyperdense left renal lesion (*red ROI*) is an enhancing mass and it has a more steeply increasing slope at lower energies. (Courtesy of Prof. Luca Volterrani, Department of Radiology University of Siena, Italy)

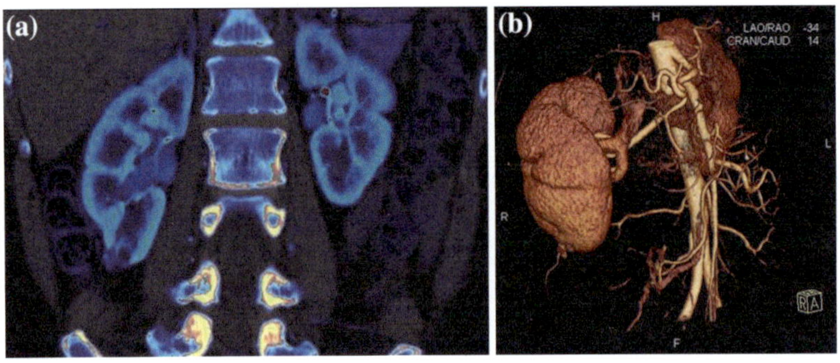

Fig. 3.20 Small cystic hypervascular renal cell carcinoma of the lower right kidney pole suitable for nephron-sparing surgery. Coronally reformatted dual-energy color-coded iodine overlay CT image during corticomedullary phase (**a**) and Volume Rendering image after dual-energy bone removal (**b**) show an accessory artery for the right lower pole and a large vein draining the tumor, both representing useful information for the surgeon

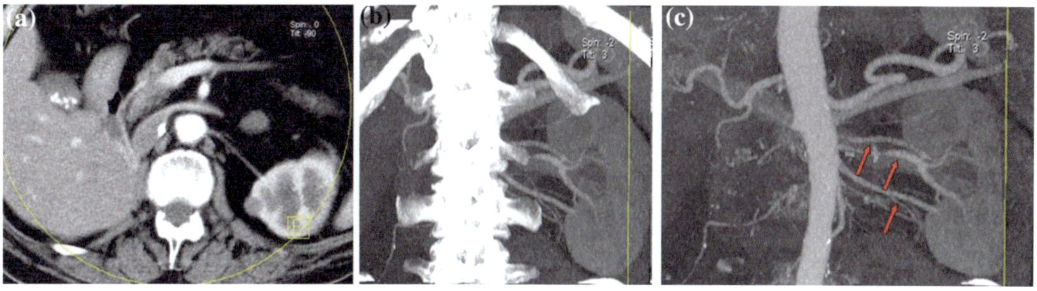

Fig. 3.21 Dual-energy linear-blended axial CT image during cortico-medullary phase (**a**) shows a small hypovascular left renal cell carcinoma in a patient with right nephrectomy. (**b**) MIP coronal CT image and (**c**) MIP coronal CT image after dual-energy bone removal. The presence of three left renal arteries, well demonstrated after bone removal (*arrows*), represents very useful pre-surgical information when a nephron-sparing surgery is expected

phase should be considered. By taking advantage of greater iodine conspicuity at 80 kVp and automated bone subtraction with the dual-energy software, effective 3D reconstruction of the renal vascular map, which are required for pre-surgical urologic planning, can be rapidly achieved (Figs. 3.20 and 3.21). The coverage of the dual-energy CT scan varies from hepatic dome to iliac crest for the corticomedullary phase, whereas from hepatic dome to pubic symphysis for the nephrographic phase.

References

1. Tada S, Yamagishi J, Kobayashi H et al (1983) The incidence of simple renal cysts by computed tomography. Clin Radiol 34:437–439
2. Jayson M, Sanders H (1998) Increased incidence of serendipitously discovered renal cell carcinoma. Urology 51:203
3. Konnak JW, Grossman HB (1985) Renal cell carcinoma as an incidental finding. J Urol 134:1094–1096
4. Luciani LG, Cestari R, Tallarigo C (2000) Incidental renal cell carcinoma-age and stage characterization and clinical implications: study of 1092 patients (1982–1997). Urology 56:58–62
5. Israel GM, Bosniak MA (2005) How I do it: evaluating renal masses. Radiology 236:441–450
6. Siegel R, Ward E, Brawley O et al (2011) Cancer statistics, 2011. CA Cancer J Clin 61:212–236
7. Lopez-Beltran A, Scarpelli M, Montironi R et al (2006) 2004 WHO Classification of the Renal Tumors of the Adults. Eur Urol 49:798–805
8. Grignon DJ, Che M (2005) Clear cell renal cell carcinoma. Clin Lab Med 25:305–316
9. Eble JN, Sauter G, Epstein JI et al (2004) Pathology and genetics. Tumors of the urinary system and male genital organs. IARC Press, Lyon
10. Brunelli M, Eble JN, Zhang S et al (2005) Eosinophilic and classic chromophobe renal cell carcinomas have similar frequent losses of multiple chromosomes from among chromosomes 1, 2, 6, 10, and 17, and this pattern of genetic abnormality is not present in renal oncocytoma. Mod Pathol 18: 161–169
11. Mostofi FK, Davis CJ (1998) Histological typing of kidney tumors. Springer, Berlin
12. Wagner BJ, Wong-You-Cheong JJ, Davis CJ Jr (1997) Adult renal Hamartomas. Radiographics 17:155–169
13. Bosniak MA (1986) The current radiological approach to renal cysts. Radiology 158:1–10
14. Harisinghani MG, Maher MM, Gervais DA (2003) Incidence of Malignancy in Complex Cystic Renal Masses (Bosniak Category III): Should Imaging-Guided Biopsy Precede Surgery? AJR 180: 755–758
15. Sauk SC, Hsu MS, Margolis DJ et al (2011) Clear cell renal cell carcinoma: multiphasic multidetector CT imaging features help predict genetic karyotypes. Radiology 261:854–862
16. Israel GM, Bosniak MA (2008) Pitfalls in Renal Mass Evaluation and How to Avoid Them. Radiographics 28:1325–1338
17. Birnbaum BA, Jacobs JE, Ramchandani P (1996) Multiphasic renal CT: comparison of renal mass enhancement during the corticomedullary and nephrographic phases. Radiology 200:753–758
18. Cohan RH, Sherman LS, Korobkin M et al (1995) Renal masses: assessment of corticomedullary-phase and nephrographic-phase CT scans. Radiology 196:445–451

19. Herts BR, Coll DM, Novick AC et al (2002) Enhancement characteristics of papillary renal neoplasms revealed on triphasic helical CT of the kidneys. AJR Am J Roentgenol 178:367–372
20. Israel GM, Silverman SG (2011) The incidental renal mass. Radiol Clin N Am 49:369–383
21. Bosniak MA (1997) Diagnosis and management of patients with complicated cystic lesions of the kidney. AJR Am J Roentgenol 169:819–821
22. Israel GM, Bosniak MA (2003) Follow-up CT of moderately complex cystic lesions of the kidney (Bosniak category IIF). AJR Am J Roentgenol 181:627–633
23. Israel GM, Bosniak MA (2003) Calcification in cystic renal masses: is it important in diagnosis? Radiology 226:47–52
24. Bosniak MA (1997) The use of the Bosniak classification system for renal cysts and cystic tumors. J Urol 157:1852–1853
25. Bosniak MA (1991) Difficulties in classifying cystic lesion of the kidney. Urol Radiol 13:91–93
26. Bosniak MA (1993) Problems in the radiologic diagnosis of renal parenchymal tumors. Urol Clin North Am 20:217–230
27. Bosniak MA (1991) The small (less than or equal to 3.0 cm) renal parenchymal tumor: detection, diagnosis, and controversies. Radiology 179:307–317
28. Hartman DS, Davis CJ, Johns T et al (1986) Cystic renal cell carcinoma. Urology 28:145–153
29. Murad T, Komaiko W, Oyasu R et al (1991) Multilocular cystic renal cell carcinoma. Am J Clin Pathol 95:633–637
30. Bosniak MA (1996) Cystic renal masses: a reevaluation of the usefullness of the Bosniak Classification System (letter). Acad Radiol 3:981–984
31. Silverman SG, Israel GM, Herts BR et al (2008) Management of the incidental renal mass. Radiology 249:16–31
32. McGahan JP, Lamba R, Fisher J et al (2011) Is Segmental Enhancement Inversion on Enhanced Biphasic MDCT a Reliable Sign for the Noninvasive Diagnosis of Renal Oncocytomas? AJR Am J Roentgenol 197:W674–W679
33. Millet I, Curros Doyon F, Hoa D et al (2011) Characterization of Small Solid Renal Lesions: Can Benign and Malignant Tumors Be Differentiated With CT? AJR Am J Roentgenol 197:887–896
34. Bosniak MA, Megibow AJ, Hulnick DH et al (1988) CT diagnosis of renal angiomyolipoma: the importance of detecting small amounts of fat. AJR Am J Roentgenol 151:497–501
35. Inzaki M, Tanimoto A, Narimatsu Y et al (1997) Angiomyolipoma: imaging findings in lesions with minimal fat. Radiology 205:497–502
36. Birnbaum BA, Hindman N, Lee J et al (2007) Renal cyst pseudoenhancement: influence of multidetector CT reconstruction algorithm and scanner type in phantom model. Radiology 244:767–775
37. Maki DD, Birnbaum BA, Chakraborty DP et al (1999) Renal cyst pseudoenhancement: beam-hardening effects on CT numbers. Radiology 213:468–472
38. Fornaro J, Leschka S, Hibbeln D et al (2011) Dual- and multi-energy CT: approach to functional imaging. Insights imaging 2:149–159
39. Johnson TR, Krauss B, Sedlmair M et al (2007) Material differentiation by dual energy CT: initial experience. Eur Radiol 17:1510–1517
40. Petersilka M, Bruder H, Krauss B et al (2008) Technical principles of dual source CT. Eur J Radiol 68:362–368
41. Graser A, Johnson TR, Chandarana H et al (2009) Dual energy CT: preliminary observations and potential clinical applications in the abdomen. Eur Radiol 19:13–23
42. Fletcher JG, Takahashi N, Hartman R et al (2009) Dual-energy and dual-source CT: is there a role in the abdomen and pelvis? Radiol Clin North Am 47:41–57
43. Kaza R, Caoili EM, Cohan RH et al (2011) Distinguishing enhancing from nonenhancing renal lesions with fast kilovoltageswitching dual-energy CT. AJR Am J Roentgenol 197:1375–1381
44. Brown CL, Hartman RP, Dzyubak OP et al (2009) Dual-energy CT iodine overlay technique for characterization of renal masses as cyst or solid: a phantom feasibility study. Eur Radiol 19: 1289–1295
45. Megibow AJ Sahani D (2012) Best practice: implementation and use of abdominal dual-energy CT in routine patient care. AJR Am J Roentgenol 199:S71–S77
46. Eusemann C, Holmes DR III, Schmidt B (2008) Dual energy CT: how the best blend both energies in one fused image? SPIE 6918 Medical imaging, San Diego
47. Kim KS, Lee JM, Kim SH et al (2010) Image fusion in dual energy computed tomography for detection of hypervascular liver hepatocellular carcinoma: phantom and preliminary studies. Invest Radiol 45:149–157
48. Yu L, Primak AN, Liu X et al (2009) Image quality optimization and evaluation of linearly mixed images in dual-source, dual-energy CT. Med Phys 36:1019–1024
49. Holmes DR, 3rd, Fletcher JG, Apel A, et al. (2008) Evaluation of non-linear blending in dual-energy computed tomography. Eur J Radiol 68:409–413
50. Apel A, Fletcher JG, Fidler JL et al (2011) Pilot multi-reader study demonstrating potential for dose reduction in dual energy hepatic CT using non linear blending of mixed kV image datasets. Eur Radiol 21:644–652
51. Ascenti G, Krauss B, Mazziotti S et al (2012) Dual-energy computed tomography (DECT) in renal masses: nonlinear versus linear blending. Acad Radiol 19:1186–1193
52. Graser A, Becker CR, Staehler M et al (2010) Single-phase dual-energy CT allows for characterization of renal masses as benign or malignant. Invest Radiol 45:399–405

53. Graser A, Johnson TR, Hecht EM et al (2009) Dual-energy CT in patients suspected of having renal masses: can virtual nonenhanced images replace true nonenhanced images? Radiology 252:433–440
54. Ascenti G, Mazziotti S, Mileto A et al (2012) Dual-source dual-energy CT evaluation of complex cystic renal masses. AJR Am J Roentgenol 199:1026–1034
55. Heye T, Nelson RC, Ho LM et al (2012) Dual-energy CT applications in the abdomen. AJR Am J Roentgenol 199:S64–S70
56. Neville AM, Gupta RT, Miller CM et al (2011) Detection of renal lesion enhancement with dual-energy multidetector CT. Radiology 259:173–183
57. Ascenti G, Mileto A, Gaeta M et al (2013) Single-phase dual-energy CT urography in the evaluation of haematuria. Clin Radiol 68:87–94
58. Kang SK, Kim D, Chandarana H (2011) Contemporary imaging of the renal mass. Curr Urol Rep 12:11–17
59. Chandarana H, Megibow AJ, Cohen BA et al (2011) Iodine quantification with dual-energy CT: phantom study and preliminary experience with renal masses. AJR Am J Roentgenol 196:693–700
60. Ascenti G, Mileto A, Krauss B, et al. (2013) Distinguishing enhancing from nonenhancing renal masses with dual-source dual-energy CT: iodine quantification versus standard enhancement measurements. Eur Radiol doi:10.1007/s0030-013-2811-4
61. Liu XL, Zhou JJ, Zeng MS et al (2013) Homogeneous high attenuation renal cysts and solid masses—differentiation with single phase dual energy computed tomography. Clin Radiol 68:198–205
62. Karlo C, Lauber A, Gotti RP et al (2011) Dual-energy CT with tin filter technology for the discrimination of renal lesion proxies containing blood, protein, and contrast-agent. An experimental phantom study. Eur Radiol 21:385–392
63. Jung DC, Oh YT, Kim MD et al (2012) Usefulness of the virtual monochromatic image in dual-energy spectral CT for decreasing renal cyst pseudoenhancement: a phantom study. AJR Am J Roentgenol 199:1316–1319
64. Yamada S, Ueguchi T, Ukai I et al (2012) The potential of dual-energy virtual monochromatic imaging in reducing renal cyst pseudoenhancement: a phantom study. Nihon Hoshasen Gijutsu Gakkai Zasshi 68:1379–1384
65. Yu L, Leng S, McCollough CH (2012) Dual-energy CT-based monochromatic imaging. AJR Am J Roentgenol 199:S9–S15
66. Silva AC, Morse BG, Hara AK et al (2011) Dual-energy (spectral) CT: applications in abdominal imaging. Radiographics 31:1031–1046

CT Urography

4

Achille Mileto, Carmelo Sofia, Silvio Mazziotti, Alfredo Blandino, Emanuele Scribano and Giorgio Ascenti

4.1 Introduction

Hematuria can have a wide range of causes, including calculi, neoplasms, infection, trauma, drug toxicity, coagulopathy, and pelvic varices. Occasionally, the cause is revealed by a clinical history of prolonged exercise or by recent instruments. Assessment for urologic malignancy is probably the most important reason for evaluating these patients; therefore, examinations with a high sensitivity for the detection of neoplasms are essential. The ability to detect other possible causes of hematuria is also important [1–3].

Many imaging modalities have been used in the evaluation of patients with hematuria.

Nowadays, cross-sectional imaging techniques, including ultrasonography (US), computed tomography (CT), and magnetic resonance imaging (MRI), have, for many indications, rapidly supplanted conventional excretory urography (EU), which has been for many decades the primary method for the imaging evaluation of the upper urinary tract [4–6].

However, initially the application of CT in the evaluation of the urothelium was somewhat limited by poor depiction of the renal collecting system and ureters due to various factors, including limited longitudinal resolution, poor urinary tract distention, and obscuration of the urothelium by dense excreted contrast medium [7]. Advances in CT technology, in particular the advent of MDCT and optimization of protocol design, have overcome these issues. Early studies in the 2000s have shown that it is possible to combine the benefits of conventional EU with those of cross-sectional imaging into a single CT study termed "CT urography," which depicts both the renal parenchyma and the whole collecting system [8–11].

Currently, typical CT urography protocols require multiple image acquisitions to obtain the unenhanced, contrast-enhanced nephrographic and excretory phases (Fig. 4.1) [1–3, 7]. Unenhanced images are useful to visualize parenchymal calcification (nephrocalcinosis), urinary calculi, hydronephrosis due to obstructing ureteral stones or urothelial tumors, hemorrhage, and infection of the urinary tract that raise urine CT attenuation and to assist in the characterization of renal masses [1–3]. Renal parenchymal abnormalities, particularly masses, are best visualized on nephrographic phase images, which also provide excellent evaluation of the other abdominal organs. Excretory phase images obtained from the kidneys to the bladder demonstrate the urinary tract distended with contrast material and are useful in detecting papillary/calyceal abnormalities as well as urothelial disease [1, 11, 12]. Although CT may also demonstrate bladder disease, flat tumors of the bladder are unlikely to be identified with CT, and cystoscopy remains the study of choice in evaluating for bladder malignancy.

In light of these applications, CT is recognized as the most sensitive and specific test for the diagnosis of urinary calculi (Fig. 4.2), renal masses, and urothelial lesions (Fig. 4.3).

G. Ascenti et al., *CT of the Retroperitoneum*,
DOI: 10.1007/978-88-470-5469-1_4, © Springer-Verlag Italia 2014

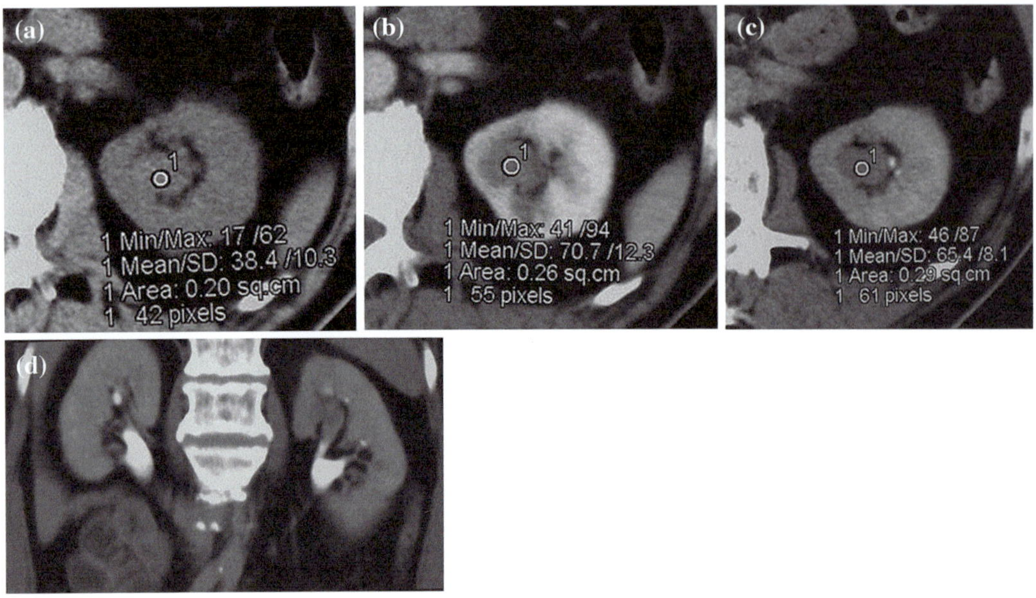

Fig. 4.1 Standard MDCT urography protocol, consisting of unenhanced (**a**), contrast-enhanced nephrographic- (**b**), and excretory phase (**c**) images, with corresponding coronally reformatted reconstruction, in a patient with urothelial lesion arising from the left kidney upper calyx. On unenhanced image (**a**), the lesion shows soft tissue attenuation and it is barely visible; a moderate contrast enhancement is seen on nephrographic phase image (**b**). On excretory phase image (**c**, **d**), the lesion is clearly visible as filling defect within the renal pelvis filled with dense contrast medium

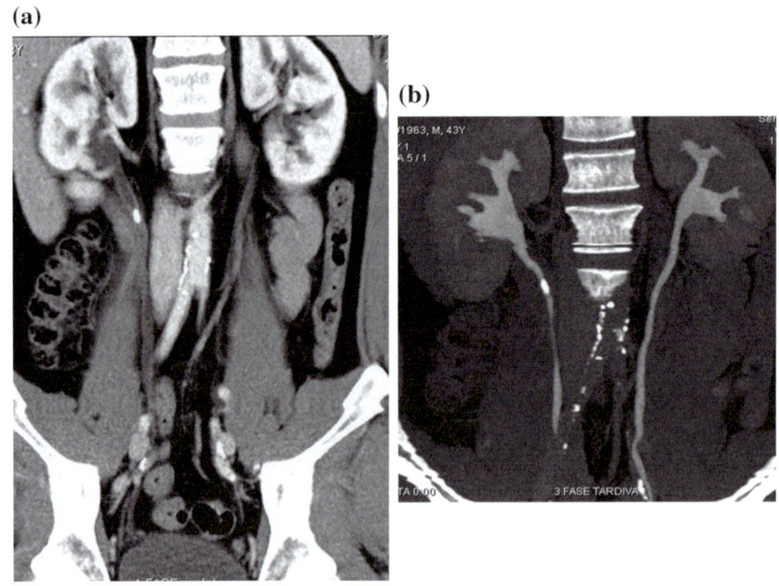

Fig. 4.2 Coronally reformatted CT images in a patient having a non-obstructing stone located in the *upper right* ureter. A mild hydronephrosis with non-obstructing stone is seen on contrast-enhanced parenchymal phase image (**a**). Simultaneous excretion of contrast medium, with no further dilatation of the right ureter, is seen on excretory phase image (**b**)

However, the principal disadvantage of CT urography is that there is an increased patient radiation dose associated with the technique; with attention to detail and judicious use of patient selection protocols, the radiation dose should be minimized. So, the outstanding question is essentially whether there are categories of patients for whom the increased sensitivity and

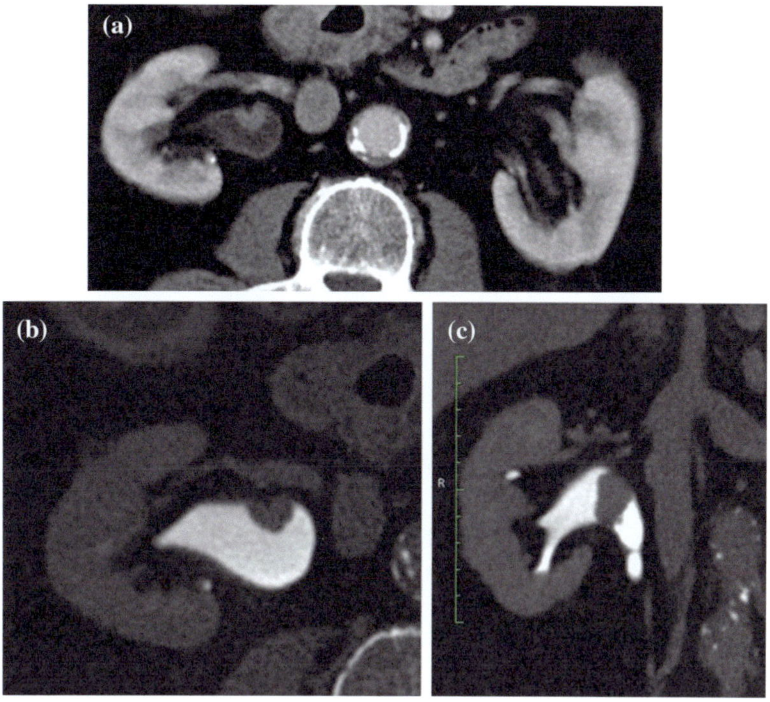

Fig. 4.3 Axial and coronally reformatted contrast-enhanced nephrographic- and excretory phase images in a patient with urothelial lesion of the right renal pelvis. A moderately enhancing vegetans lesion is seen on axial contrast-enhanced nephrographic phase image (**a**). On axial (**b**) and coronally reformatted (**c**) excretory phase images, the lesion is clearly visible as filling defect within the renal pelvis full of dense contrast medium

specificity of CT urography justify the increased radiation dose. The obvious category comprises those patients with suspected urological cancer and, in particular, patients whose own risk factors for urological malignancy include increasing age (>40 years), smoking, macroscopic compared with microscopic hematuria (4:1), and exposure to aniline dyes. In these patients, a reasonable strategy to limit radiation dose exposure is considering CT urography as the final step of the urologic evaluation, always and only after the patient undergoes urinalysis and cystoscopy.

4.2 State of the Art of Conventional (Multidetector) CT

MDCT urography is today recognized as state-of-the-art imaging modality in the evaluation of hematuria. It allows fast and high-resolution volumetric scanning of the urinary tract in a single comprehensive examination, termed "*one-stop-shop modality,*" offering several three-dimensional post-processing features including multi-planar reformations (MPR) and maximum intensity projection (MIP) images (Fig. 4.4) [1–3, 7].

For most of the different CT urographic techniques, no special preparation is necessary. Oral hydration (usually 500–700 ml of water to drink in the waiting room) and voiding before starting the examination of the patient are two basic pre-requirements for CT urography. In many centers, in order to achieve an optimal distension of the excretory system and to dilute iodine contrast medium otherwise too dense, a diuretic-enhanced CT urography technique is performed with the additional injection of low-dose furosemide (between 5 and 10 mg, i.e., an individual dose of 0.1 mg furosemide per kg of body weight) before the beginning of CT examination. Several studies have demonstrated that the use of low-dose diuretics provide benefits for obtaining accurate depiction of the urinary tract morphology and fine anatomic details, such as calyceal fornices visualization (Fig. 4.5) [1, 13].

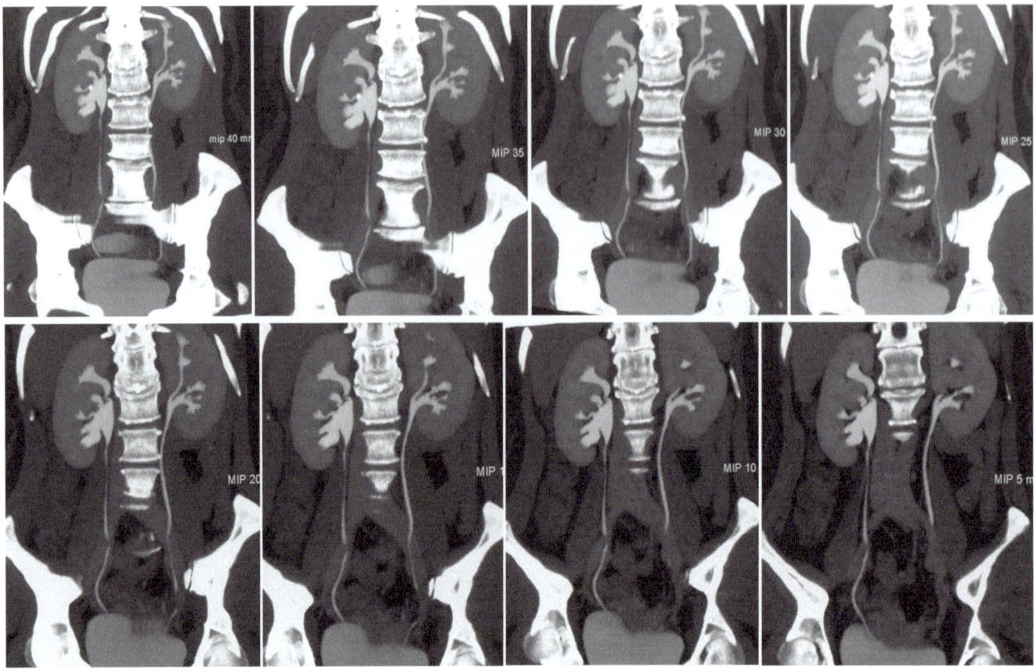

Fig. 4.4 Coronally reformatted MIP images at different thickness (40–5 mm) in a patient with *left* Bertin's column hypertrophy and associated double renal collecting system

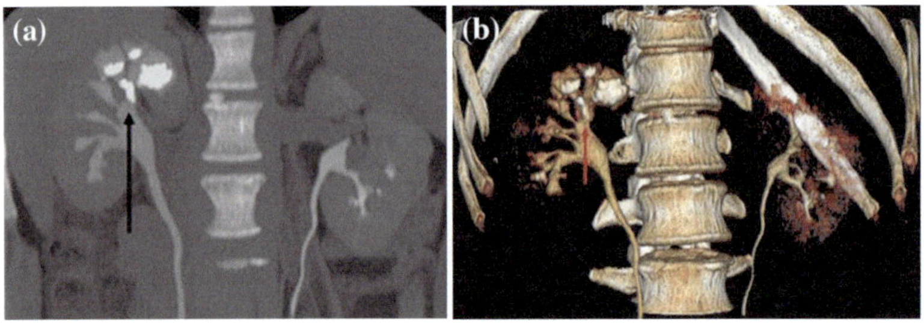

Fig. 4.5 Coronally reformatted excretory phase image with corresponding VRT image in a patient with intrarenal calculosis (*arrow*). Both excretory images provide an accurate depiction of the urinary tract morphology and calyceal fornices visualization

The first step of CT urography examination is always unenhanced acquisition, from the upper renal pole to the pubic symphysis. In particular, care has to provide on the topogram to include the entire bladder. Afterward, as with conventional excretory urography, a single intravenous bolus of contrast medium is usually administered in CT urography, as well. The volume of the contrast material bolus ranges from 100 to 150 ml, administered at a rate of 2–3 ml/sec [1, 3, 7, 10, 11, 13].

Any urographic imaging technique presupposes at least one data acquisition during the excretory phase. Thus, some authors simply use a single-phase CT urographic protocol [14]. However, in the common sense, to exploit all the potential of this technique, CT urography is understood as a combination of renal CT plus

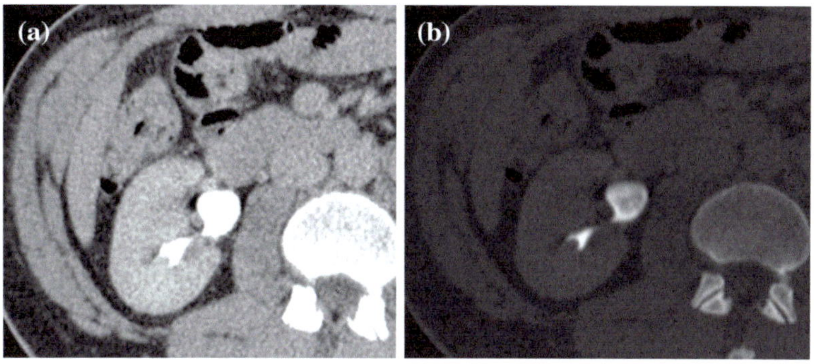

Fig. 4.6 Axial excretory phase images with different windowing levels in a patient with urothelial tumor of the right renal pelvis. Note that soft tissue window setting (**a**) is highly affected from noise and dense endoluminal contrast material hides the presence of subtle alterations, whereas a wide window setting (**b**) offers an almost noise-free evaluation of urothelium and calyceal details

CT of the contrast-enhanced upper urinary tract. Therefore, in most centers, a three-phase CT urographic protocol, consisting of unenhanced, nephrographic, and excretory phases, is performed [1, 3, 7].

During any CT urography acquisition protocol, some tricks, such as abdominal compression ("compression CT urography") or the injection of a saline chaser bolus, to improve the distension of the upper urinary tract can be adopted [15–17]. Some authors suggest that a significant improvement in the opacification of the middle and distal ureters on the post-release excretory phase scan is achieved, whereas other authors report that no significant difference in ureteral distension exists on CT urography without compression. Several studies have utilized intravenous saline chaser injection technique [15, 16]. As diuretic-enhanced CT urography technique, supplemental hydration may improve the distension of the urinary tract by increasing the urine volume, but also causes endoluminal dilution of the excreted amount of contrast material. Several studies found a significant improvement in the opacification of the pelvicalyceal system and the proximal ureters [15–17]. However, the opacification of the middle and distal ureteral segments does not profit significantly from saline chaser injection [1].

An alternative to the single-bolus injection technique with subsequent three-phase acquisition protocol is represented by the "split-bolus CT urography". Using the split-bolus technique, one injects initially only 40–50 ml of contrast medium. After a delay of several minutes (generally 6–7 min), another 80–110 ml of contrast material is administered, and then, a CT scan is obtained after a delay of 90–100 s. The split-bolus technique generates a combined nephrographic and pyelographic phase, which allows for a simultaneous assessment of the renal parenchyma in the nephrographic phase and the pelvicalyceal system in the excretory phase by acquisition of only a single CT scan. In particular, with first bolus of contrast medium, urinary excretion of contrast medium is achieved, whereas the renal nephrogram is obtained with the second bolus [1, 18, 19].

MDCT urography usually produces about 300–700 slices per series, making workstation review mandatory. Axial images, reconstructed with a thickness of 5 mm, are for the most part sufficient for diagnosis and MPR images used for display. Many authors recommend wide window settings for the evaluation of the urothelium and calyceal details on excretory phase images, because artifacts from dense endoluminal contrast material are less disturbing (Fig. 4.6) [1, 3, 19]. Tiny neoplastic lesions lying in the axial plane are hard to identify on axial images, so MPR review is generally recommended [20–26]. From the excretory phase multi-slice volumetric dataset, thin-slab or thick-slab maximum intensity projection (MIP) images and volume

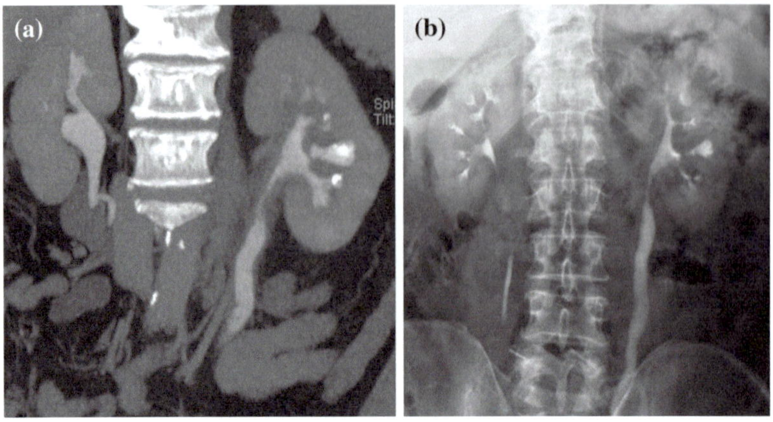

Fig. 4.7 Coronally reformatted contrast-enhanced excretory phase image (**a**) with corresponding conventional urogram image (**b**) in a patient with infiltrating urothelial lesion of the left renal pelvis

rendering (VR) images can be reconstructed to obtain typical urographic views similar to conventional urograms (Fig. 4.7).

As one may guess, numerous different examination techniques exist to put MDCT urography into operation, including various ways in administering the contrast agent and achieving complete urinary tract opacification. However, while a substantial homogeneity in diagnostic performances between different CT urography protocols exists, they are dramatically heterogeneous with each other in terms of radiation dose exposure [1, 3, 27–29].

In conventional EU, the delivered effective radiation dose was usually between 1.5 and 4 mSv, depending on acquisition parameters, number of films acquired, patient size and gender. With three- or two-phase CT urography approach, mean effective doses of 20.1 mSv, approximately 5 times higher than those of excretory urography, have been reported. Even, for a four-phase CT urography protocol, the calculated average effective dose is between 25 and 35 mSv [27–32]. Consequently, in the evaluation of patients with a high pretest probability of malignant urothelial disease, the "*As Low As Reasonably Achievable* (ALARA)" principle should always be kept in mind. In order to contain the radiation dose, the first strategy is to reduce the number of study phases and the scanning coverage. Based on the specific clinical context (e.g., proven urothelial disease), a dual-phase (unenhanced and excretory phases) protocol can be carried out. Adopting the split-bolus technique may represent an optimal compromise to not preclude the possibility of a renal parenchyma evaluation even though the patient does not have a high pretest probability of renal neoplastic disease [1, 18, 19].

More recently, several technologies that are available on commercial CT systems are geared toward radiation dose reduction by a scanning parameters modulation. Dose management technology in CT has led to optimization of CT protocols using angular (x and y-axes), longitudinal (z-axis), or combined (x, y, and z-axes) modulation of the dose; in some modern systems, this can also be combined with 3D adaptive noise filtration [1, 11, 12].

However, current studies are moving in the direction of performing CT urography using a low-tube-voltage dual-energy CT urography with synchronous nephrographic/excretory enhancement. One study demonstrated that the diagnostic quality of low-tube-voltage (80 kVp) excretory phase images is comparable with that of 120-kVp images. Given the significantly lower radiation dose (greater than 50 %) and greater opacification of the urinary system with low-tube-voltage (80 kVp) images, the use of 80-kVp images in the excretory phase of CT urography seems to be feasible. However, this approach is problematic in terms of increased image noise and applicability, especially in the US population due to higher BMI values.

4.3 Spectral CT: Study Protocols and Clinical Applications

The advent of dual-energy CT represents a unique opportunity for CT urography to significantly reduce the radiation dose while ensuring high diagnostic performances.

By exploiting the difference in CT attenuation of different materials as a function of electron densities and photon energies, it allows the identification, separation, and quantification of certain material compositions [33–36]. If materials having sufficiently different *K*-edges, defined as "*a sudden increase in attenuation at photon energy levels just above the K-shell binding energy*," are shown at two different energies (80/100 and 140 kVp), they can be characterized on the basis of variations in photon absorption at different photon energies (e.g., calcium or iodine can be distinguished from soft tissues based on their differences in K-edges) [33–35, 37]. In light of this basic physical assumption, iodinated contrast medium can be completely subtracted to obtain virtual unenhanced images and one of the main purposes of unenhanced images during CT urography (i.e., urinary calculi detection) could be achieved without requiring an unenhanced scan, therefore significantly cutting the radiation dose exposure [33, 36, 37].

In daily clinical practice, urinary stone detection as well as pre- and post-contrast HU attenuation measurement on the upper and lower urinary tract is crucial to evaluate patients with hematuria, hydronephrosis, urinary tract tumors, congenital anomalies, chronic urolithiasis, and patients' pre- and post-surgical status. In order to fully omit standard unenhanced acquisition, the first issue deserving to be addressed is whether urinary stones can be detected by means of high-attenuating iodinated contrast medium subtraction from the renal parenchyma or whether collecting system and virtual unenhanced images provide reliable CT attenuation measurements [38].

With the use of a phantom model, one study showed the dual-energy CT iodine subtraction virtual unenhanced technique is capable of depicting urinary stones submerged in iodine solutions [38]. Subsequent clinical studies also demonstrated that virtual unenhanced images reconstructed from nephrographic phase scans are helpful for detecting urinary stones with a sensitivity of 83 and 63 % [39, 40]. All the studies found that most stones appear slightly smaller or less conspicuous on virtual unenhanced images than on the true unenhanced images (Fig. 4.8). This is due to subtraction of some stone signal from the stone periphery along with the iodine signal. In addition, the difference in collimation between dual-energy (1.2 mm) and single-energy (0.6 mm) acquisitions determines a relatively

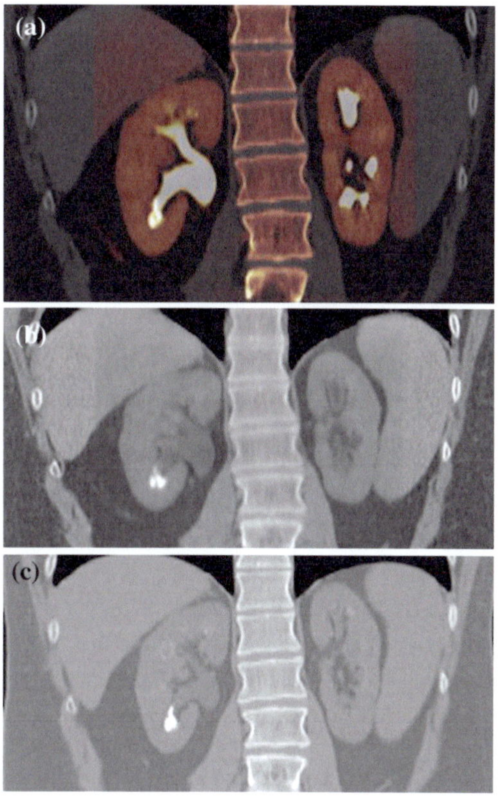

Fig. 4.8 Coronally reformatted dual-energy color-coded iodine overlay image with simultaneous nephrographic/excretory enhancement (**a**), corresponding virtual unenhanced image, obtained after spectral-based iodine subtraction (**b**), and standard unenhanced single-energy image (**c**). Virtual unenhanced image (**b**) depicts intrarenal calculosis as well as standard unenhanced single-energy image (**c**) does. However, note that stones are less conspicuous on virtual unenhanced image (**b**) compared to standard unenhanced single-energy image (**c**)

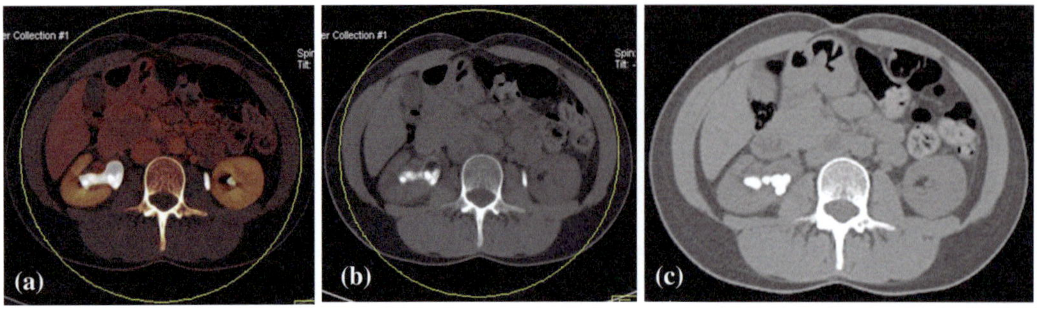

Fig. 4.9 Axial dual-energy color-coded iodine overlay image with simultaneous nephrographic/excretory enhancement (**a**), corresponding virtual unenhanced image, obtained after spectral-based iodine subtraction (**b**), and standard unenhanced single-energy image (**c**). Compared to standard unenhanced single-energy image (**c**), a good iodine spectral extraction is achieved for the posterior right renal pelvis with subsequent depiction of stones. However, the very dense iodine in the urine led to an excessive iodine subtraction for the anterior right renal pelvis with a signal void artifact; the lack of iodine subtraction in the left proximal ureter is also seen

lower *z*-axis resolution that does not allow separation of the small stones and iodine in the urinary tract because of the volume averaging [41–43]. Similar results have been reported by reconstructing virtual unenhanced images from synchronous nephrographic/excretory enhancement (split-bolus CT urography technique) dual-energy CT images [44]. Furthermore, in all these studies, it emerged that the presence of very dense iodine in the urine leads to insufficient or excessive subtraction of contrast medium (Fig. 4.9). In particular, a recent study showed that highly concentrated iodine causes a breakdown of the iodine subtraction algorithm [38].

All these initial clinical experiences in dual-energy CT urography had been carried out with the use of a first-generation dual-source dual-energy CT scanner. Due to an energy spectra overlap between 100 and 140 kVp, these scanners had to be operated at 80 and 140 kVp, resulting in the inability to be used in the abdomen due to a low penetration depth and beam-hardening artifact [40, 41].

The introduction of a second-generation dual-source dual-energy scanner overcame these issues. On this dual-energy hardware platform, a tin filtration (a selective photon shield) of the high-energy (140 kVp) spectrum, labeled with the acronym "*140 kVp (Sn)*," dramatically reduces the X-ray spectra overlap with CT attenuation values close to the standard unenhanced images and narrows the 140-kVp X-ray spectrum which entails better radiation dose efficiency and less beam-hardening artifacts [42, 43].

A phantom experiment, performed with a second-generation dual-source dual-energy system, demonstrated that the implementation of high-energy X-ray spectrum tin filtration permits to lower at 730 HU the breakdown point of iodine subtraction algorithm in very dense iodinated solution; at attenuation levels higher than 730 HU, beam hardening begins to influence the iodine CT value in the low kV and high kV images, resulting in an increasingly inaccurate virtual unenhanced image inside the volume of the iodine container [45]. A more recent clinical study showed that after virtual elimination of contrast medium, while large and high-attenuation stones can be reliably detected, smaller and lower attenuation calculi might be erased from images, especially with increased image noise [43, 46]. Thus, in the clinical use of virtual unenhanced images at the excretory phase of CT urography, this pitfall should be taken into account.

The possibility of reconstructing virtual unenhanced images from dual-energy contrast-enhanced data has the potential to revive CT urography that still today remains a "radiation-intensive study." From a clinical point of view, the advantages of spectral-based iodine extraction with subsequent creation of virtual unenhanced images can be maximally exploited if a split-bolus CT urography injection/acquisition technique is carried out (Fig. 4.10) [36, 44, 46, 47].

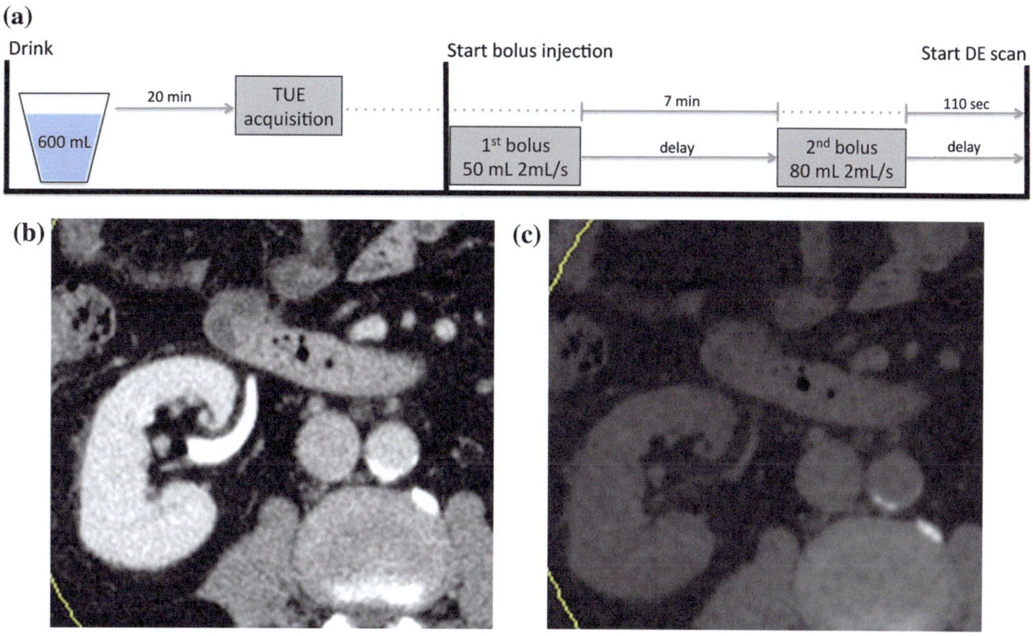

Fig. 4.10 Example of split-bolus dual-energy MDCT urography protocol (**a**) and corresponding acquired datasets, consisting of contrast-enhanced image with simultaneous nephrographic/excretory enhancement (**b**) and virtual unenhanced image (**c**) obtained by means of spectral-based iodine subtraction

The simultaneous nephrographic parenchymal contrast enhancement and urographic excretion allow the radiologist to detect urinary stones or parenchymal calcification on virtual unenhanced images, to characterize renal lesions by means of color-coded display of the iodine distribution in the scan field, and to identify urothelial lesions. Until now, at least two- or three-phase CT urography protocols were needed to achieve these three main clinical tasks; dual-energy CT urography with synchronous nephrographic/excretory enhancement represents an "all-in-one" approach that accurately enables this in a single-phase CT acquisition, with subsequent dramatic reduction in terms of radiation dose exposure. Recent studies showed that a radiation dose saving up to 50 % can be achieved by means of a single-phase CT urography with synchronous nephrographic/excretory enhancement (split-bolus CT urography technique) [44, 46, 47].

Finally, dual-energy CT urography was found to be accurate enough in the specific setting of urothelial tumor identification (Fig. 4.11). One recent study [35] showed that dual-energy CT urography with synchronous nephrographic/excretory enhancement had a sensitivity of 85.7 %, a specificity of 98.6 %, a positive predictive value of 92.3 %, and a negative predictive value of 97.1 % for urothelial tumor detection [35]. This study raised the problem that single-phase split-bolus dual-energy CT urography does not permit in most cases an adequate opacification of the lower urinary tract [44]. In addition to well-known MDCT spatial resolution limits, single-phase split-bolus dual-energy CT urography is not an optimized injection protocol for the lower urinary tract. There is thus the risk to overlook pretty tiny or flat urothelial lesions, especially those located in the lower ureters or in the bladder. Although conventional cystoscopy undoubtedly remains the gold standard for evaluation of the lower urinary tract urothelium and patients with hematuria should ideally undergo conventional cystoscopy before CT urography, the possibility to add a low-dose single-energy acquisition to a split-bolus CT urography protocol should be taken into account. In this setting, a careful

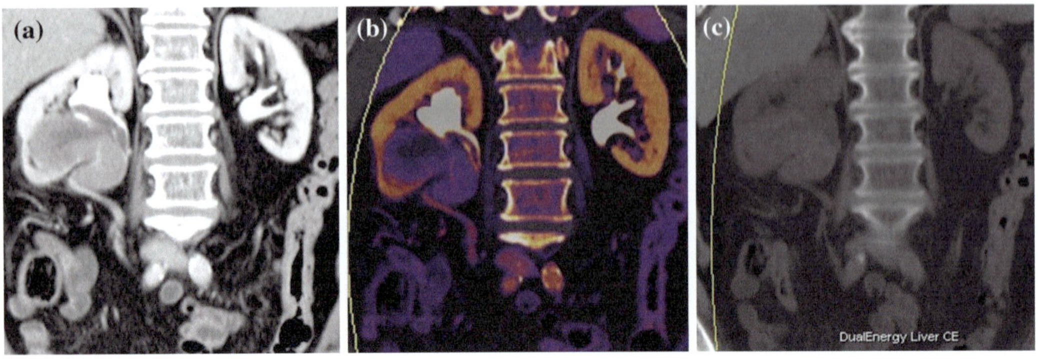

Fig. 4.11 Coronally reformatted dual-energy image with simultaneous nephrographic/excretory enhancement (**a**), corresponding color-coded iodine overlay (**b**) and virtual unenhanced image (**c**) in a patient with urothelial mass of the right renal pelvis. Note that compared with grayscale image (**a**), color-coded iodine overlay image (**b**) provides benefits in distinguishing between the solid enhancing and the necrotic component of the mass. Virtual unenhanced image (**c**) shows a clinically acceptable image quality

balance between radiation dose and image quality should be made and, above all, tailored to the specific clinical context. The combination of different injection techniques and the adjunct of saline bolus chaser to currently used protocols may represent a future field of investigation that might broaden the clinical feasibility of dual-energy CT urography without sacrificing radiation dose saving.

References

1. Nolte-Ernsting C, Cowan N (2006) Understanding multislice CT urography techniques: many roads lead to Rome. Eur Radiol 16:2670–2686
2. Chai RY, Saini S, Hahn PF, Mueller PR (2000) Comprehensive "one-stop" evaluation of patients with haematuria using multi-slice CT. Radiology 217:454–455
3. Van Der Molen AJ, Cowan NC, Mueller-Lisse UG et al (2008) CT urography: definition, indications and techniques. A guideline for clinical practice. Eur Radiol 18:4–17
4. Amis ES (1999) Epitaph for the urogram. Radiology 213:639–640
5. Grossfeld GD, Litwin MS, Wolf JS et al (2001) Evaluation of asymptomatic microscopic hematuria in adults: the American Urological Association best practice policy–part II: patient evaluation, cytology, voided markers, imaging, cystoscopy, nephrology evaluation, and follow-up. Urology 57:604–610
6. Joffe SA, Servaes S, Okon S et al (2003) Multi–detector row CT urography in the evaluation of hematuria. Radiographics 23:1441–1456
7. Perlman ES, Rosenfield AT, Wexler JS et al (1996) CT urography in the evaluation of urinary tract disease. J Comput Assist Tomogr 20:620–626
8. Caoili EM, Inampudi P, Cohan RH et al (2003) MDCTU of upper tract uroepithelial malignancy. AJR Am J Roentgenol 180:71
9. Caoili EM, Cohan RH, Korobkin M et al (2002) Urinary tract abnormalities: initial experience with multi-detector row CT urography. Radiology 222:353–360
10. McCarthy CL, Cowan NC (2002) Multidetector CT urography (MDCTU) for urothelial imaging. Radiology 225(Suppl):237
11. McTavish JD, Jinzaki M, Zou KH et al (2002) Multi-detector row CT urography: comparison of strategies for depicting the normal urinary collecting system. Radiology 225:783–790
12. Tsili AC, Efremedis SC, Kalef-Ezra J et al (2007) Multidetector-row CT urography on a 16-row CT scanner in the evaluation of urothelial tumors. Eur Radiol 17:1046–1054
13. Kemper J, Regier M, Stork A et al (2006) Improved visualization of the urinary tract in multidetector CT urography (MDCTU): analysis of individual acquisition delay and opacification using furosemide and low-dose test images. J Comput Assist Tomogr 30:751–757
14. Girish G, Agarwal SK, Salim F et al (2003) Single-phase multislice CT urography: initial experience. Eur Radiol 13:147
15. Caoili EM, Inampudi P, Cohan RH et al (2005) Optimization of multi- detector row CT urography: effect of compression, saline administration, and prolongation of acquisition delay. Radiology 235:116–123
16. Chow LC, Sommer FG (2001) Multi-detector CT urography with abdominal compression and three-dimensional reconstruction. AJR 177:849–855

17. Sudakoff GS, Dunn DP, Hellman RS et al (2006) Opacification of the genito- urinary collecting system during MDCT Urography with enhanced CT digital radiography: nonsaline versus saline bolus. AJR Am J Roentgenol 186:122–129
18. Chow LC, Kwan SW, Olcott EW et al (2007) Split bolus MDCT urography with synchronous nephrographic and excretory phase enhancement. AJR Am J Roentgenol 189:314–322
19. Korobkin M (2005) CT urography. Eur Radiol 15:s82–s84
20. Bosniak MA (1991) The small (less than or equal to 3.0 cm) renal parenchymal tumor: detection, diagnosis, and controversies. Radiology 179:307–317
21. Hartman DS, Davis CJ, Johns T et al (1986) Cystic renal cell carcinoma. Urology 28:145–153
22. Murad T, Komaiko W, Oyasu R et al (1991) Multilocular cystic renal cell carcinoma. Am J Clin Pathol 95:633–637
23. Bosniak MA (1996) Cystic renal masses: a reevaluation of the usefulness of the Bosniak Classification System (letter). Acad Radiol 3:981–984
24. Silverman SG, Israel GM, Herts BR et al (2008) Management of the incidental renal mass. Radiology 249:16–31
25. McGahan JP, Lamba R, Fisher J et al (2011) Is Segmental Enhancement Inversion on Enhanced Biphasic MDCT a Reliable Sign for the Noninvasive Diagnosis of Renal Oncocytomas? AJR Am J Roentgenol 197:W674–W679
26. Millet I, Curros Doyon F, Hoa D et al (2011) Characterization of Small Solid Renal Lesions: can Benign and Malignant Tumors Be Differentiated With CT? AJR Am J Roentgenol 197:887–896
27. Kemper J, Begemann PGC, Regier M et al (2005) Multislice-CT-urography (MSCTU): experimental evaluation of low-dose protocols. Eur Radiol 15:273
28. Kalra MK, Maher MM, Rizzo S et al (2004) Radiation exposure and projected risks with multidetector-row computed tomography scanning: clinical strategies and technologic developments for dose reduction. J Comput Assist Tomogr 28:S46–S49
29. Greess H, Wolf H, Baum U et al (2000) Dose reduction in computed tomography by attenuation-based on-line modulation of tube current: evaluation of six anatomical regions. Eur Radiol 10:391–394
30. Vrtiska TJ, Hartman RP, Kofler JM et al (2009) Spatial resolution and radiation dose of a 64-MDCT scanner compared with published CT urography protocols. AJR 192:941–948
31. McCollough CH, Bruesewitz MR, Vrtiska TJ et al (2001) Image quality and dose comparison among screen-film, computed, and CT scanned projection radiography: applications to CT urography. Radiology 221:395–403
32. Shinagare AB, Sahni VA, Sadow CA et al (2011) Feasibility of low tube voltage excretory phase images during CT urography: assessment using a dual-energy CT scanner. AJR Am J Roentgenol 197:1146–1151
33. Johnson TR, Krauss B, Sedlmair M et al (2007) Material differentiation by dual energy CT: initial experience. Eur Radiol 17:1510–1517
34. Graser A, Johnson TR, Chandarana H et al (2009) Dual energy CT: preliminary observations and potential clinical applications in the abdomen. Eur Radiol 19:13–23
35. Fletcher JG, Takahashi N, Hartman R et al (2009) Dual-energy and dual-source CT: is there a role in the abdomen and pelvis? Radiol Clin North Am 47:41–57
36. Hartman R, Kawashima A, Takahashi N et al (2012) Applications of dual- energy CT in urologic imaging: An update. Radiol Clin North Am 50:191–205
37. Petersilka M, Bruder H, Krauss B et al (2008) Technical principles of dual source CT. Eur J Radiol 68:362–368
38. Takahashi N, Hartman RP, Vrtiska TJ et al (2008) Dual-energy CT iodine-subtraction virtual unenhanced technique to detect urinary stones in an iodine-filled collecting system: a phantom study. AJR Am J Roentgenol 190:1169–1173
39. Scheffel H, Stolzmann P, Frauenfelder T et al (2007) Dual-energy contrast-enhanced computed tomography for the detection of urinary stone disease. Invest Radiol 42:823–829
40. Takahashi N, Vrtiska TJ, Kawashima A et al (2010) Detectability of urinary stones on virtual nonenhanced images generated at pyelographic-phase dual-energy CT. Radiology 256:184–190
41. Primak AN, Giraldo JC, Eusemann CD et al (2010) Dual-source dual-energy CT with additional tin filtration: Dose and image quality evaluation in phantoms and in vivo. AJR Am J Roentgenol 195:1164–1174
42. Primak AN, Ramirez Giraldo JC, Liu X et al (2009) Improved dual-energy material discrimination for dual-source CT by means of additional spectral filtration. Med Phys 36:1359–1369
43. Mangold S, Thomas C, Fenchel M et al (2012) Virtual nonenhanced dual-energy CT urography with tin-filter technology: determinants of detection of urinary calculi in the renal collecting system. Radiology 264:119–125
44. Ascenti G, Mileto A, Gaeta M et al (2013) Single-phase dual-energy CT urography in the evaluation of haematuria. Clin Radiol 68:87–94
45. Toepker M, Moritz T, Krauss B et al (2012) Virtual non-contrast in second- generation, dual-energy computed tomography: reliability of attenuation values. Eur J Radiol 81:398–405
46. Karlo CA, Gnannt R, Winklehner A et al (2013) Split-bolus dual energy CT urography: protocol optimization and diagnostic performance for the detection of urinary stones. Abdom Imaging. doi: 10.1007/s00261-013-9992-9
47. Takeuchi M, Kawai T, Ito M et al (2012) Split-bolus CT-urography using dual-energy CT: feasibility, image quality and dose reduction. Eur J Radiol 81:3160–3165

Urinary Stones

5

Achille Mileto, Bernhard Krauss, Silvio Mazziotti,
Alfredo Blandino, Carmelo Sofia and Giorgio Ascenti

5.1 Introduction

Nephrolithiasis is a worldwide problem, sparing no geographical, cultural, or racial groups [1–3]. The prevalence of urinary stones has progressively increased in industrialized nations, and a similar trend is being observed in developing countries due to changing social and economic conditions [1–4]. In the USA, approximately 1.2 million people are affected annually, and it is estimated that up to 14 % of men and 6 % of women will develop stone disease during their lifetime [1, 5]. In addition, many patients will be affected by multiple stones throughout their lifetime, with estimated recurrence rates of 50 % within 5–10 years and 75 % within 20 years [1, 6–8]. The rising prevalence of urinary stone disease has had a significant impact on the healthcare system due to the direct costs involved and the morbidity associated with complications such as infection and chronic renal failure [6–8].

Wide geographical variations exist in stone incidence and composition, and regional stone belts have been identified, where raised incidence has been attributed to genetic and environmental factors, such as hot climate (fluid loss) and sun exposure (vitamin D) [8]. Kidney stones are composed of inorganic and organic crystals amalgamated with proteins. Crystallization and subsequent lithogenesis can happen with many solutes in the urine. Calcareous stones are still by far the most common nephroliths, accounting for more than 80 % of stones [1, 3–5]. Uric acid stones represent about 5–10 %, trailed by cystine, struvite, and ammonium acid urate stones (Fig. 5.1). Miscellaneous types of highly uncommon stones are associated with xanthine, 2, 8-dihydroxyadenine, protein matrix, and drugs—e.g., indinavir and triamterene. Stones of mixed composition are not uncommonly encountered [1, 3–5]. A pure uric acid versus a uric acid-containing calcium oxalate stone might show quite different underlying pathophysiologies, such as the presence of hypercalciuria [1].

There are several conditions that can contribute to the formation of kidney stones [1, 9]. The urine supersaturation is of great importance in the understanding of kidney stones pathophysiology. Since the concentration rather than the amount of the crystallizing solutes is what ultimately establishes stone formation, reduced urinary volume will amplify the saturation of all solutes and raise the risk of all stone formations [1, 9]. When high concentrations of stone-forming substances such as calcium oxalate, calcium phosphate, or struvite are present in the urine, one or more crystals may form and become trapped within the urinary tract. The crystal may attract other crystals and bind together with them, growing into a stone. Another important factor contributing to stone formation is an uneven balance of acid in the urine [1, 9, 10]. The acidity or alkalinity of the urine affects the ability of stone-forming substances to remain dissolved. Some types of stones will only form in acidic urine; others will form only in alkaline urine.

G. Ascenti et al., *CT of the Retroperitoneum*,
DOI: 10.1007/978-88-470-5469-1_5, © Springer-Verlag Italia 2014

Fig. 5.1 Frequency and chemical composition of renal stones

Stone type (chemical composition)	Frequency (%)
Calcium oxalate-monohydrate	40-60
Calcium oxalate-dehydrate	40-60
Calcium phosphate (apatite; Ca10[PO4]6[OH]2)	20-60
Calcium phosphate (brushite; CaHPO4·2H2O)	2-4
Uric acid	5-10
Struvite (magnesium ammonium phosphate)	5-15
Cystine	1.0-2.5
Ammonium urate	0.5-1.0
Mixed calcium oxalate-phosphate	35-40
Mixed uric acid-calcium oxalate	5

Finally, the lack of substances in the urine that prevent the growth of crystals plays an important role. Normally, substances that inhibit the formation and growth of crystals, such as pyrophosphates, citrates, and magnesium, are present in the urine. A decrease or absence of these substances may cause a stone to develop [9, 10].

Renal colic is the most common clinical manifestation associated with kidney stone and is due to the anatomic progression of a stone from the renal pelvis down the ureter, with dramatic relief upon passage of the stone [1, 11, 12]. Stones that are impacted at the ureteropelvic junction produce flank pain, whereas stones lodged in the proximal ureter (between the ureteropelvic junction and the iliac vessels) cause flank pain radiating to the genitals. Stones lodged at the ureterovesical junction produce voiding urgency and suprapubic discomfort, and they cause pain that radiates into the groin and genitals. Associated symptoms include gross or microscopic hematuria, nausea, and vomiting [1, 11, 12].

Nephrolithiasis can also present as a secondary complication, such as an obstruction or a urinary tract infection [1].

Concomitant with the increasing prevalence of urolithiasis is the growing utilization of imaging for diagnosis, treatment planning, and post-treatment follow-up. Imaging in urolithiasis has evolved over the years due to technologic advances and a better understanding of the disease process. While in the past standard radiography and intravenous urography have played a pivotal role in the diagnosis and treatment of patients with acute ureterolithiasis, since its introduction in the early 1990s, unenhanced CT has become the modality of choice in kidney stones imaging [11, 12].

5.2 State of the Art of Conventional (Multidetector) CT

Unenhanced CT has emerged as the diagnostic imaging modality of choice for the evaluation of suspected renal colic and has proved useful in the pre-therapeutic assessment of urinary tract stones [11–17].

Since the first description of its utility by Smith et al. in 1995 [18], unenhanced CT has been found to have a high degree of sensitivity (95–98 %) and specificity (96–100 %) in the diagnosis of urolithiasis [12, 19–23]. CT has several advantages over other imaging techniques: it can be performed rapidly, does not require the administration of contrast material, is highly sensitive for the detection of stones of all sizes, and allows for the detection of alternative causes of flank pain [12, 19–22]. Appendicitis, diverticulitis, pancreatitis, and gynecologic lesions are often detected by CT in patients with non-specific abdominal pain mimicking ureteral colic when the diagnosis may not be obvious prior to imaging [12]. An additional benefit of CT is its ability to reveal urinary congenital abnormalities, infections, and neoplasms, whose diagnoses have a greater clinical relevance than that of stone disease [12].

The introduction of MDCT in 1998 has opened up new prospects for CT imaging of kidney stones [11, 12]. Thanks to acquisition of isotropic volume and three-dimensional evaluation of these isotropic data sets, radiologists have been empowered to meet the greater expectations of urologists in the assessment of stone disease [12, 19–24]. The identification of the number, size, and location of calculi and determination of the presence of hydronephrosis (i.e., obstruction) are routinely made with MDCT. High-resolution coronally reformatted images generated automatically from isotropic data sets obtained with 16–64-detector CT allow more rapid and accurate detection of urinary stones than axial images alone [12, 19–24].

The scanning technique and parameters for unenhanced multidetector CT for urolithiasis should be tailored toward the indication. It is also important to keep in mind that a CT protocol for the evaluation of stone disease is not considered equivalent to routine unenhanced abdominopelvic CT [12, 19–23]. The former should typically include scanning of the entire urinary tract from the upper pole of the kidneys to the base of the urinary bladder. Although bladder distention has been recommended for enhanced visualization of distal ureteral stones, the improved accuracy of multidetector CT due to the availability of coronally reformatted images usually obviates any patient preparation [12, 19–23].

Thin (1–3 mm) reconstruction sections are recommended for better detection and characterization of urinary calculi, particularly small stones, due to the reduction in partial volume averaging effect. Acquiring CT scans with a section thickness greater than 5 mm can lead to frequent missing of small urinary calculi and can also affect size and attenuation measurements, due to partial volume averaging effect resulting in lower average values [10, 12, 25]. Virtually, all stones are of sufficient attenuation to be revealed on CT including those that are radiolucent on conventional radiographs, such as uric acid, xanthine, and cystine stones [11]. These stones have an attenuation value (>200 HU) greater than that of the surrounding soft tissue, and multidetector CT helps accurately localize a stone within the renal pelvicaliceal system or ureter. The only known exception is a stone that consists entirely of protease inhibitors, such as indinavir sulfate (Crixivan; Merck, Rahway, NJ), used in the treatment for human immunodeficiency virus infection [12, 26].

The most reliable CT sign for ureterolithiasis is a stone within the ureteral lumen, with proximal ureteral dilatation and a normal distal caliber (Fig. 5.2).

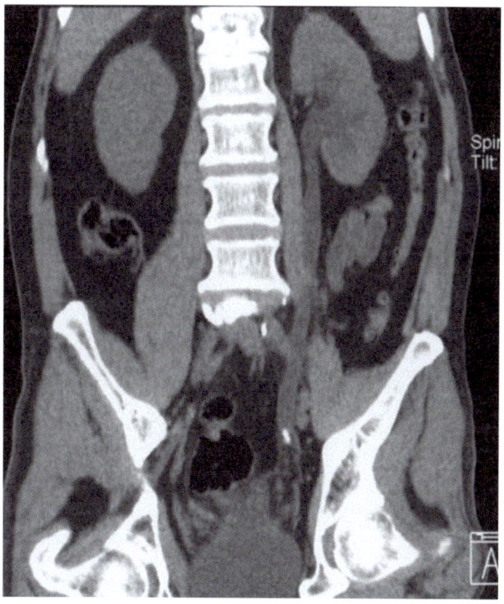

Fig. 5.2 Coronally reformatted unenhanced CT image in a patient with left flank pain permits direct visualization of a small stone located in the lower left ureter with proximal dilatation and normal distal ureteral caliber

In addition to the direct visualization of a stone in the lumen of the ureter, the diagnosis of ureterolithiasis can be confirmed on the basis of several secondary signs by CT as well. The most reliable signs include hydronephrosis, perinephric and periureteral stranding/edema, and unilateral renal enlargement [12]. Ureteral dilatation has a sensitivity of approximately 90 % for use in making a diagnosis of acute ureteral obstruction. Similarly, stranding of the perinephric and periureteral fat has sensitivities of approximately 85 % [12, 27]. In the subgroup of patients with acute flank pain, the presence of both ureteral dilatation and perinephric stranding has a positive predictive value of nearly 100 %, and the absence of both findings has a negative predictive value of approximately 95 % for the diagnosis of acute ureterolithiasis [12, 27].

Less reliable findings include unilateral absence of the white renal pyramid, thickening of the lateroconal fascia, and differences in renal parenchymal attenuation between obstructed and non-obstructed kidneys [12, 27].

One common pitfall in the interpretation of unenhanced CT is the confusion of a phlebolith with a ureteral stone, especially in the pelvis. Therefore, differentiation between stones and other calcific processes is an important issue. Two signs, the "soft tissue rim sign" and the "comet tail sign," have been described for the differentiation of ureteral stones from these calcifications [12, 27]. The "soft tissue rim sign" consists of a soft tissue attenuation halo around a calcific focus and is very specific for ureteral stones rather than phleboliths [12, 27, 28]. The "soft tissue rim" represents the edematous wall of the ureter around the stone and has a sensitivity of 50–77 % and a specificity of 90–100 % [12, 28]. The presence or absence of the rim is found to correlate with the size of the stone rather than the degree of obstruction [12, 27, 28]. The "comet tail sign" is created by an eccentric, tapering soft tissue area adjacent to the calcification and is a reliable feature in the diagnosis of phleboliths (Fig. 5.3). Another feature that is helpful in differentiation is the central lucent area seen in phleboliths, in contrast to the opacified centers seen in stones [12, 27, 28].

Once the diagnosis of obstruction by a ureteral stone has been made on CT, prognosis and patient treatment can be guided on the basis of CT findings. Stone burden evaluation at CT is one of the most important factors in determining treatment strategies and management in cases of urolithiasis [12]. Ege et al. [27] reported that stones greater than 6 mm in diameter in the proximal ureter accompanied by more than five secondary signs of obstruction are more likely to necessitate intervention such as endoscopic removal or lithotripsy than those with fewer secondary signs. Novel semiautomatic segmentation tools can also be used to estimate stone volume, which has been shown to be valuable for preoperative planning [12].

Today, multidetector CT is faced with two "burning issues": the radiation dose to patients and stone composition characterization.

The problem of radiation dose is of particular concern in young individuals who undergo repeated CT examinations due to recurrent stone disease and is consequently likely to be at risk for greater cumulative lifetime exposure [12, 29–33]. Numerous practical approaches for dose reduction in CT for urolithiasis have been advocated in the literature [12, 30–36]. Implementation of strategies targeted at dose reduction at every step of the CT protocol can considerably reduce the radiation dose for each CT examination. One strategy consists of the use of low-dose multidetector CT protocols in which the tube current and tube potential are appropriately lowered [12, 29–36]. Use of very low tube current (50–100 mAs) compared with that used for diagnostic examinations can offer radiation dose reduction of up to 80 % while maintaining diagnostic performance for stone detection [12, 29–36]. An accuracy of 93–97 % has been achieved in the detection of urinary calculi with these low-dose techniques [12, 29–33]. However, the use of these techniques with a fixed tube current is not suitable for patients of different sizes. Rather, the scanning technique must be customized to the patient's size [12, 37].

Other recently advanced solutions to minimize the radiation dose are automatic tube current modulation technique and iterative image

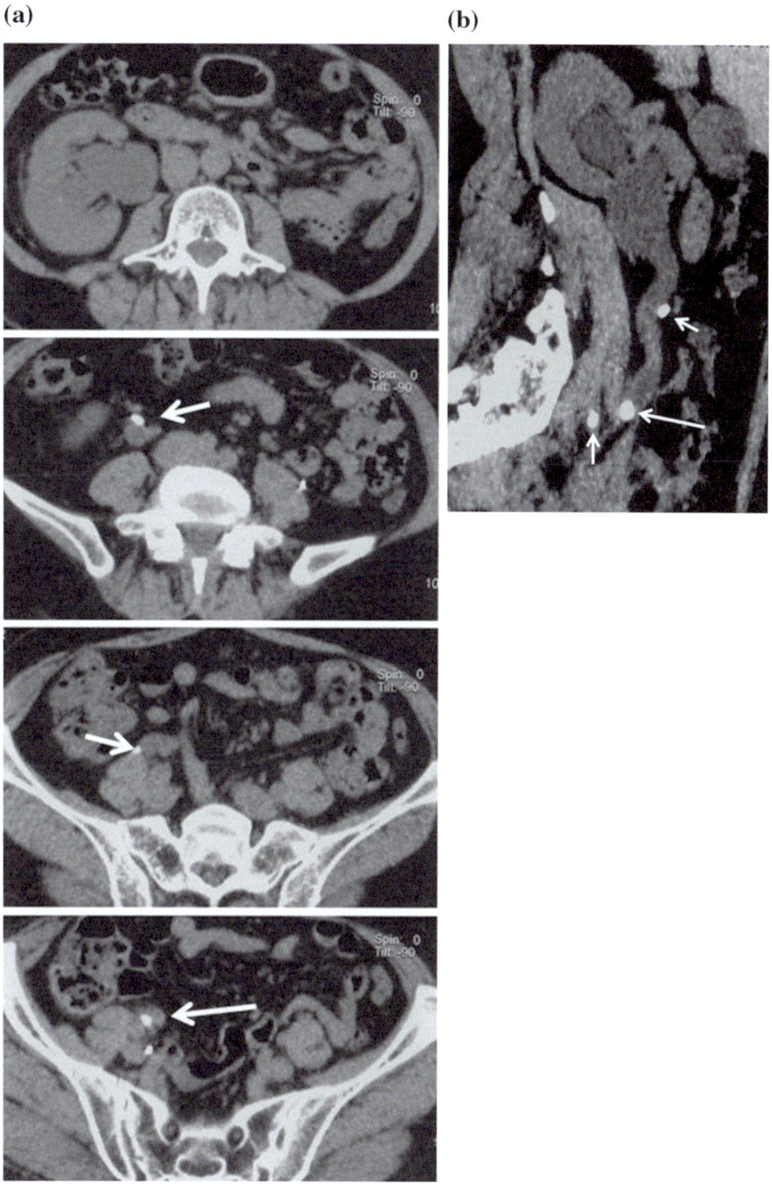

Fig. 5.3 Right ureteral calcolosis with hydronephrosis and multiple phleboliths. Unenhanced axial CT images (**a**) show right hydronephrosis due to the presence of an iliac ureteral stone. The "soft tissue rim sign" is well appreciated (*arrow*). Many calcifications close to the ureter are due to phleboliths (*short arrows*). Parasagittally reformatted CT image (**b**) easily distinguish the intraureteral stone (arrow) from phleboliths (*short arrows*)

reconstruction algorithms. By modulating noise index and reference milliamperage, it is possible to achieve the objective of radiation dose reduction. However, this technique is problematic in terms of high noise levels, which can cause severe graininess of images and impact accuracy in the diagnosis of small calculi [12, 37]. Iterative image reconstruction algorithm has been recently introduced for MDCT scanners with the goal of reducing image noise [38, 39]. In an iterative reconstruction, a correction loop is introduced into the image generation process [38, 39]. Synthesized projection data are compared to real measurement data in an iterative manner: the update image is refreshed by a correction image, and prior knowledge is imposed on image data. Compared with standard computed filtered back-projection technique, iterative reconstructions permit to acquire CT data at lower radiation dose level while maintaining a higher level of image quality [38, 39].

The other critical issue MDCT has to face with are the knowledge of stone composition, as it is the key determinant of urologic appropriate management [12]. In particular, determination of stone composition is of particular importance because uric acid stones may be treated with urinary alkalinization as a first-line treatment, with surgical treatment being reserved for stones that do not respond to medical therapy, whereas stones of certain compositions (e.g., cystine stones), as well as calcium-based stones of certain attenuation, are extremely difficult to fragment with ESWL [12, 40].

The attenuation values of urinary calculi at conventional 120 kVp, usually fall within certain ranges: uric acid, 200–450 HU; struvite, 600–900 HU; cystine, 600–1100 HU; calcium phosphate, 1200–1600 HU; and calcium oxalate monohydrate and brushite, 1700–2800 HU [12, 41]. Helical CT attenuation as well as stone density can be used to predict stone composition in vitro with 64–81 % accuracy [12]. Although uric acid, cystine, calcium oxalate monohydrate, and brushite calculi have been identified in vitro with an accuracy exceeding 85 % on the basis of attenuation measurements [12, 41], the differentiation between stone types is more complicated and less reliable in vivo than in vitro. Among other factors, it is dependent on the size and accurate placement of the region of interest, it is affected by the section thickness, and MDCT is still unable to fully address this issue.

5.3 Spectral CT: Study Protocols and Clinical Applications

The X-ray attenuation of chemical compositions depends on their density, on their atomic number, and on the energy (X-ray spectrum) of the penetrating beam. The energy dependency of the attenuation is linked to the atomic number; with increasing atomic numbers of the penetrated chemical elements, the energy dependency of the attenuation also increases [42–45]. In urinary calculi, various chemical elements can be found. While calcium oxalate (CaC_2O_4), calcium phosphate ($Ca_3(PO_4)_2$), and cystine ($C_6H_{12}N_2O_4S_2$) contain elements with high atomic numbers, uric acid ($C_5H_4N_4O_3$) and struvite ($(NH_4)MgPO_4{\cdot}{}_6H_2O$) are mainly composed of elements with lower atomic numbers [42, 43, 46].

The effective atomic numbers of the uric acid stone types fall into a narrow range (approximately 6.84–7.01). The effective atomic numbers of non-uric acid stones are higher and more varied (range 10.78–15.56) [47–50]. The large difference in the effective atomic numbers of uric acid and non-uric acid stones explains the ability of dual-energy CT to differentiate uric acid from non-uric acid stones with high accuracy. However, the differences in the effective atomic numbers between the common non-uric acid stones, such as cystine, struvite, calcium oxalate, brushite, and apatite, are much smaller [51–58]. Spectral-based dual-energy CT analysis became today reliable approach to noninvasively analyze the chemical composition of urinary calculi, by interrogating the attenuation both at high and low energy levels [42–46, 59–61].

Instead of material decomposition, the dual-energy "material labeling" only distinguishes material A from material B, but does not provide the concentration of any material.

For the differentiation between several types of kidney stones, measurements of the effective atomic number or the dual-energy index (DEI) can be used [47, 62]. Measurements of the effective atomic number make use of an additional approximation to the base material decomposition approach. It is assumed that the X-ray attenuation of a material for the relevant energy range is identical to the attenuation of two other materials, that coherent scattering can be neglected, that Compton scattering is independent of the atomic number, and that the photoelectric effect is proportional to the nth power of the atomic number. The measured effective atomic number can be calculated from the true chemical composition of an object if the parameter n, which was used for image calculation, is known. The following equation is adopted to calculate the effective atomic number. The expression is then:

$$Z_{\text{eff}} = \left(\frac{\sum_i n_i Z_i^{n+1}}{\sum_i n_i Z_i} \right)^{1/n}$$

where n_i denotes the number density of the atom type i, and Z_i denotes its atomic number. For clinical dual-energy CT, the coefficient n is approximately 3. Reliability of the measured effective atomic number decreases for materials with atomic numbers over calcium, which has no limitation in the case of kidney stones.

DEI [63], which is closely related to the original CT values x_1 at low kV and x_2 at high kV is calculated using the following equation:

$$DEI = \frac{x_1 - x_2}{x_1 + x_2 + 2{,}000\,\text{HU}}$$

Both the effective atomic number and the DEI are sensitive to partial volume effect, and for small stones (<5 mm), it is potentially difficult to measure the true effective atomic number or the true DEI. The characteristic ratio, on the other hand, is by definition insensitive to this [64].

Quantities which are more stable in the presence of partial volume effects can also be used; as kidney stones are often small and surrounded by soft tissue, the effective atomic number will increase between the apparent surface and the center of a calcified stone. The characteristic ratio can overcome this problem [53, 54].

Kidney stones that are embedded in a certain soft tissue always show CT values at both energies that are between the CT values of the tissue and the CT values of the stone (Fig. 5.4).

In addition, comprehensive approaches, which use all available information at the same time to distinguish also different types of calcified stones, that have very similar dual-energy properties appear feasible [65].

First results about kidney stone composition characterization have been described using dual-source dual-energy CT platform [53–56, 61] in the differentiation between uric acid and non-uric acid renal stones (Fig. 5.5). Because uric acid calculi comprise approximately 10 % of stone disease and are typically treated medically, using urinary alkalization with stone dissolution, separating this specific subtype of stone provides a potential first management step in a renal stone treatment algorithm [57]. The dual-source dual-energy system offers a rapid characterization tool at the time of initial imaging evaluation, using a three-material decomposition algorithm that assumes every voxel includes a component of water, calcium, and/or uric acid. The voxels are then color coded based on the quantity of each of these components (Syngo Kidney Stone, Siemens AG, Forchheim, Germany). The processing time using this tool is rapid, requiring only few minutes, resulting in display of uric acid stones with a red overlay and non-uric acid with a blue overlay display (Figs. 5.5 and 5.6) [47, 48, 51–58, 66–68].

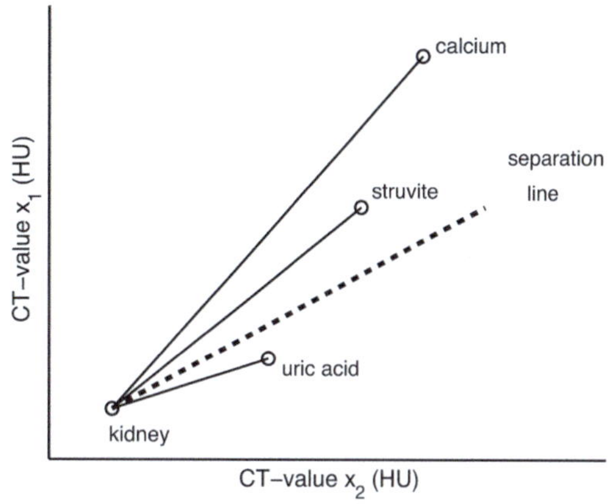

Fig. 5.4 Material labeling for kidney stones: the measured CT values of small, pure stones will be on the connecting lines between kidney and the pure stone material. The slope of the connecting line indicates the stone type

Differentiation of uric acid from non-uric acid stones was first performed using in vitro models with high sensitivity and accuracy (88–100 %) [57].

In vivo studies for kidney stone characterization also demonstrated high accuracy for differentiating uric acid and non-uric acid stones [51–57]. Separation of uric acid and non-uric acid stones has been performed using a low-dose protocol, with sensitivity of 100 % and specificity of 97 % [42].

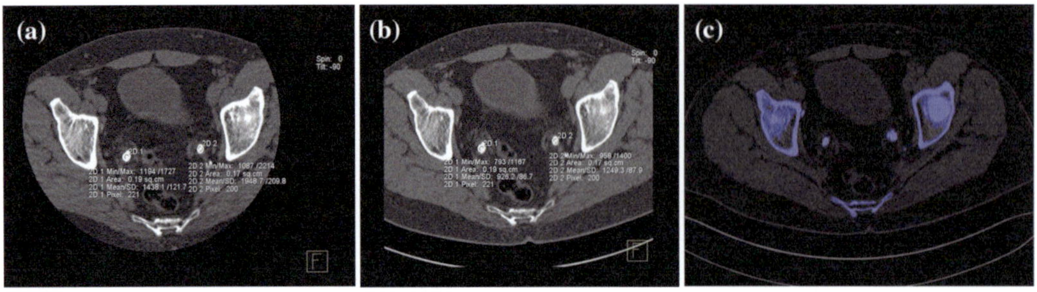

Fig. 5.5 Patient with bilateral pelvic ureteral calculosis. Dual-energy unenhanced axial CT images at 80 kVp (**a**), at 140 kVp (**b**), and color-coded image (**c**) obtained by using Kidney Stone Dual Energy software (Siemens Healthcare). Both stones presented high attenuation value at 80-kVp image (**a**) compared to the 140 kVp one (**b**). The 80 and 140 kVp Hounsfield numbers ratio is 1,55 for both stones and the system assigns a blue color indicating a non-uric acid stone composition (**c**)

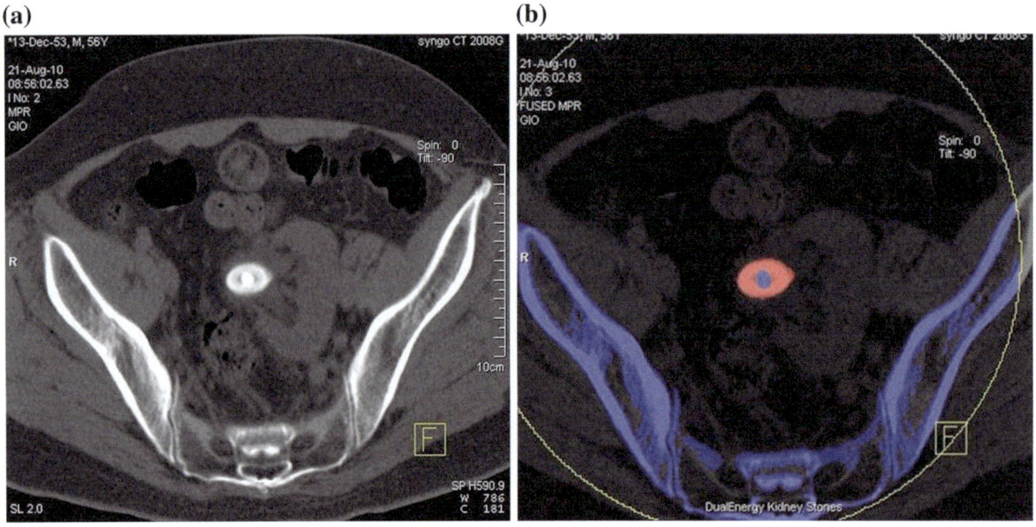

Fig. 5.6 Left ectopic, pre-sacral kidney with an oval stone in the ureteropelvic junction. Low-dose unenhanced single energy (**a**) and dual-energy color coded (**b**), obtained by using Kidney Stone software (Siemens Healthcare), axial CT images. **Panel b** shows that the stone is predominantly composed of uric acid (*red color*) with a higher attenuation calcific core (*blue color*)

Attention has to be paid if stones are closed to ureteral stents. Depending on the chemical composition, stents can be visualized as uric acid or non-uric acid [69, 70], but their high CT value can change the apparent type of nearby stones as mathematical filter algorithms may include them in the analysis of the true stone [70]. The characterization of additional stone types other than uric acid is important to patient's management, because stones known to be resistant to extracorporeal shock wave lithotripsy, including brushite, cystine, and calcium oxalate monohydrate, can be directed to management by percutaneous or endoscopic stone removal. Moreover, characterization of struvite stones directs the surgeon to total stone removal rather than allowing for small residual fragments that may result in persistent symptoms and recurrent stone growth. Boll and Ziberman [50, 56] demonstrated that a non-commercially available data processing technique with voxel-by-voxel analysis can potentially identify five unique renal stone subtypes both in vitro and in vivo (uric acid, cystine, struvite, calcium oxalate/calcium phosphate, and brushite). Accurate separation of cystine as a unique stone subtype has also been performed in vivo (Fig. 5.7) [57]. However, the ability of dual-energy CT to discriminate between two materials is highly dependent on the difference between each material's characteristic CT number ratio, which is defined as the ratio of the CT number of a given material in the low-energy image to the CT number of the same material in the high-energy image [48]. The difference between the CT number ratios for any two materials is determined by the separation between the low- and high-energy spectra and

(a)
(b)

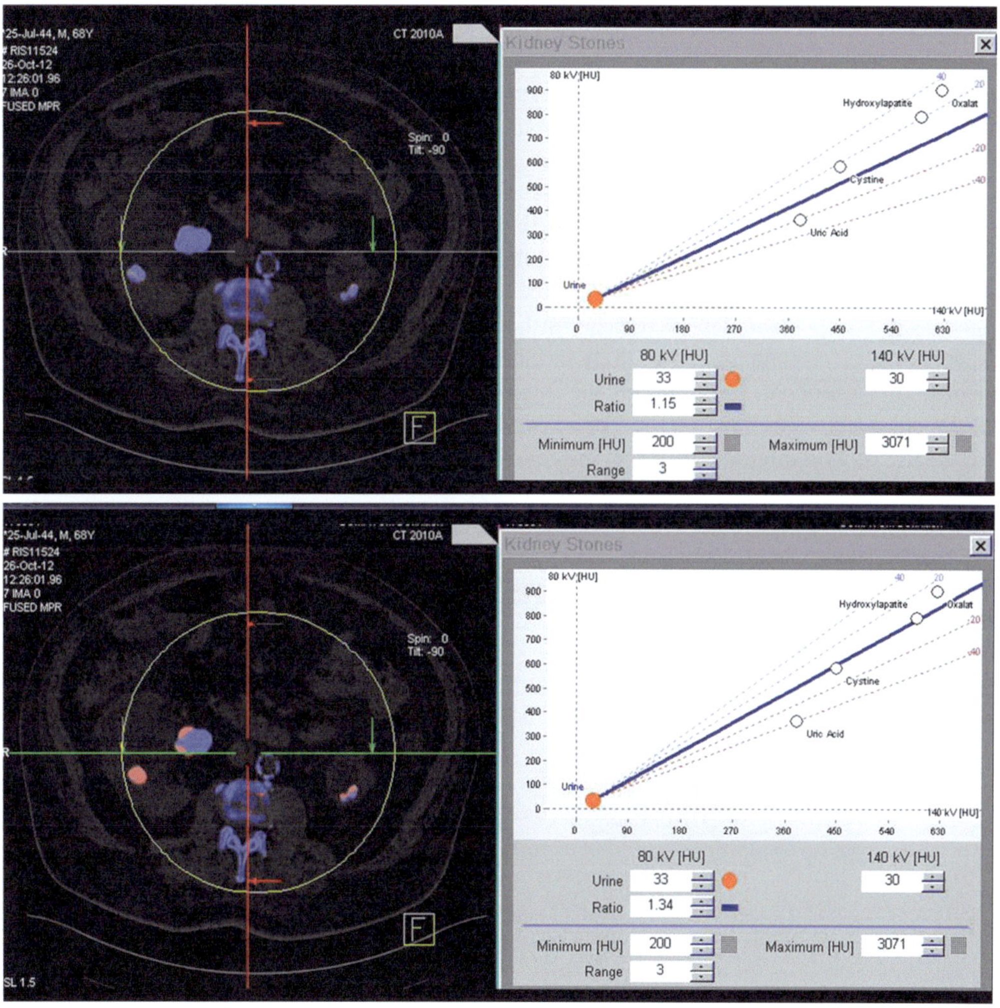

Fig. 5.7 Combined calcium and cystine stone. **a** and **b** *left panels* show axial CT images centered on stones in both kidneys. **a** and **b** *right panels* show elaboration with Kidney Stones software (Siemens Healthcare). In diagram, four stone types (hydroxyapatite, calcium oxalate, cystine, and uric acid) are described by *four small circles* (140 kVp CT density is displayed on *x-axis*, and 80 kVp CT density is displayed on *y-axis*). *Blue line* splits plane into two parts; if line is left in its default position and orientation (**a**), lower part contains non-calcium stones (cystine and uric acid) and upper part contains calcium stones (hydroxyapatite, calcium oxalate). Stones are automatically painted red by software if its CT density lies in lower part of diagram (i.e., *under line*) or blue if its CT density lies in upper part of diagram. When parameters are changed and DE ratio increased to 1,34 (**b**), blue line varies its orientation, and consequently, cystine (in red color) can be easily differentiate from calcium oxalate

the effective atomic numbers of the evaluated materials [48, 49]. The larger spectral separation, the better material discrimination is achieved, especially in the case of non-uric acid stones, which all have similar effective atomic numbers. Spectral separation can be increased by using different filtration on the two X-ray tubes [48, 49]. In the first-generation dual-source scanner (Somatom Definition DS, Siemens Healthcare), both X-ray tubes had the same filtration and the X-ray spectra generated at two different tube potentials have significant overlap [48, 49]. A phantom experiment showed that the use of additional tin filtration on the high-energy X-ray tube of a dual-source CT system operated at 80 and 140 kV can reduce the spectral overlap from 93 to 27 % and significantly improved the separation of non-uric acid stone types by CT number ratio [48]. These data have been further validated by a recent in vivo study which adopted an additional filtration of the high-energy spectrum. This investigation concluded that the use of a tin filter allows for an improved spectral separation between calcium and iodine. [48, 49]. The second-generation dual-source CT system (Somatom Definition Flash, Siemens Healthcare) has a tin filter installed on the high-energy X-ray tube to improve the X-ray spectral separation. This is able to increase the differences in the dual-energy CT number ratio between the different stone types [48, 49]. Using this new dual-source system, an ex vivo study done by Stolzmann et al. [47] showed significant improvement in differentiating uric acid from non-uric acid stones (Fig. 5.8). These experiments showed that dual-energy CT material discrimination was improved, without an increase in radiation dose, compared with single-energy CT techniques. Recently, Qu et al. [49] have demonstrated both in vitro and in vivo that second-generation dual-source dual-energy CT system with tin filtration permits to accurately distinguish up to four different classes of kidney stones, including uric acid stones, cystine stones, struvite/calcium oxalate di- or monohydrate stones, apatite stones, in a patient cohort

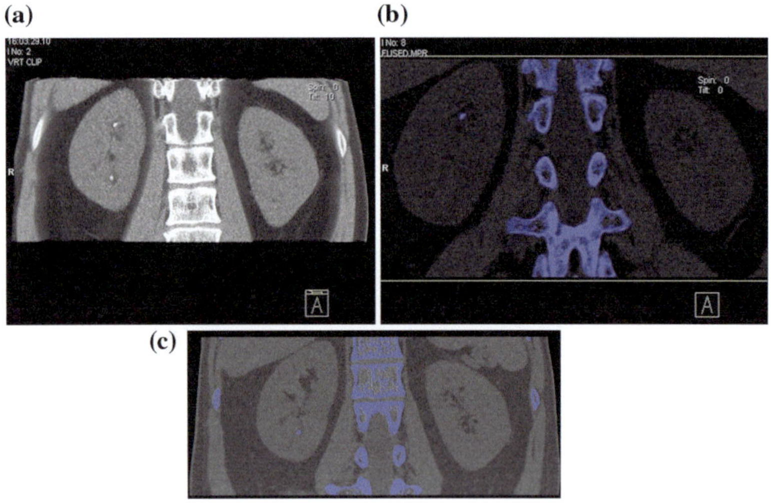

Fig. 5.8 Patient with two small stones at upper and lower right kidney calices. Coronally reformatted single-energy unenhanced VRT image (**a**) and coronally reformatted second-generation dual-energy CT images (**b**, **c**) obtained by using Kidney Stone software (Siemens Healthcare). Both are correctly depicted and characterized as non-uric acid stones (*blue color*) (**b**, **c**)

with a wide range of body habitus by the use of size-adaptive thresholds for each patient [49]. This approach provided an overall accuracy of 79.1 % for stone type characterization [48, 49]. These results are truly promising since the main drawback of first-generation dual-source system operating at 80-/140-kVp settings, is overcome. In fact, the use of a first-generation dual-source system is not recommended for larger patients due to an insufficient photon flux when the tube is operated at 80 kV. This results in excessive image noise if these patients are imaged (Fig. 5.9) [48, 49]. This is an important limitation, for example, for US patient population where the mean body mass index value is usually over 30 kg/m^2.

Table 5.1 shows different parameters for in vitro determination of renal stone composition with different DECT systems [49, 70, 71].

Initial studies demonstrate that accurate classification of mixed stone types is more challenging than pure stone types [72]. Further research is needed to depict the distinctive portions of stone disease containing more than one component.

Although the dual-energy acquisitions often do not increase the radiation dose when compared with routine single-energy acquisitions, CT examinations for kidney stones assessment, especially in the recurrent stone former, who may require multiple examinations over their lifetime, are often acquired with low-radiation-dose acquisitions [57]. Alternatively, a tailored approach to characterize urinary calculi could use a low-dose unenhanced CT of the urinary system, followed by limited unenhanced dual-energy acquisitions of the urinary tract containing a visible calculus (Fig. 5.10). In a recent study, Ascenti et al. [72] characterized 24/24 of ureteral calculi larger than 3 mm as uric acid, calcium salt, or combined uric acid–calcium salt using stone-targeted dual-energy CT with 100 % specificity. Based on in vitro measured data, this "stone-targeted" protocol reduced dose by up to 50 % compared with a full dual-energy acquisition [72].

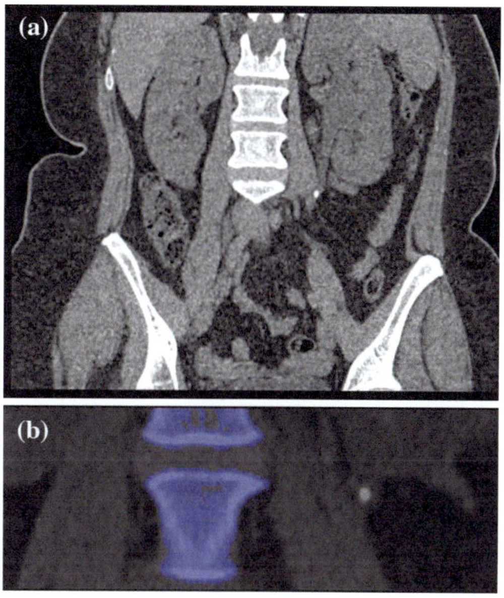

Fig. 5.9 Obese patient with a small (4 mm) left ureteral stone. Low-dose unenhanced single energy (**a**) and dual-energy (**b**), obtained by using Kidney Stone software (Siemens Healthcare), coronally reformatted CT images. Note the great noisy image at low-dose unenhanced single-energy CT scan (**a**) and the impossibility of characterizing the small calculus at first-generation DECT study

Kidney stones characterization can also be achieved on a single source with rapid kilovolt peak switching dual-energy CT hardware platform, wherein an X-ray tube capable of rapid modulation of kilovoltage and milliamperage allows switching between low (80 kVp) and high (140 kVp) energy levels [12, 58]. Unlike dual-source CT, with its image-based dual-energy processing, this technique features dual-energy processing of projection data [12]. Theoretically, this allows for accurate material decomposition and monochromatic CT image display, which should potentially facilitate more precise tissue characterization and also substantially minimize imaging artifacts [12].

Table 5.1 In vitro determination of renal stone composition with different DECT systems and parameters, after creation of stone library

Authors	Analysis	Stone composition	Parameters			DE system
Hidas G Radiology 2010	In vitro	Uric acid Cystine Calcified	<1.1 1.1–1.24 >1.24			Single-source CT Two-layer detectors
Qu M EurRadiol 2012	In vitro	Uric acid Cystine Struvite, Brushite, Caoxalate Apatite	0.98–1.01 1.15–1.24 1.26–1.37 1.32–1.45			Dual-source CT Second generation
Li XH Clinical Radiology 2013	In vitro	Uric acid Struvite Cystine Ca oxalate Ca phosphate		−3.55–1477.02 224.99–1068.51 139.67–1112 518.61–946.59 619.39–901.39	0.03 0.19 0.13 0.58 0.69	Single-source CT Fast-kVp switching
			Low kVp/ High kVp Ratio	Calcium–water density (mg/ml)	Calcium–water Ratio	

Renal stone characterization with single-source fast-kVp switching dual-energy CT platform relies on projection-space data utilization. There is the expectation that a significant improvement in stones characterization can be enabled with respect to image-domain analysis performed with the dual-source system [58]. Particularly, there is the potential to differentiate stones that are composed primarily of uric acid, calcium oxalate, cystine, or struvite. These data can be viewed as a separate display (so-called "Effective Z"), or overlaid onto the monochromatic images. For example, a calcium:uric acid material base pair image set is generated with calcium-containing calculi predominantly seen on calcium density image and uric acid-containing calculi predominantly seen on the uric acid density image [58].

Although renal stone characterization on single-source fast-kVp switching dual-energy platform is as yet a work-in-progress, preliminary investigations suggest that a multi-parametric approach using material base pairs, computed monochromatic attenuation with spectral HU curve, and effective Z analysis has potential for the discrimination of various kidney stone types [57].

(a)

(b)

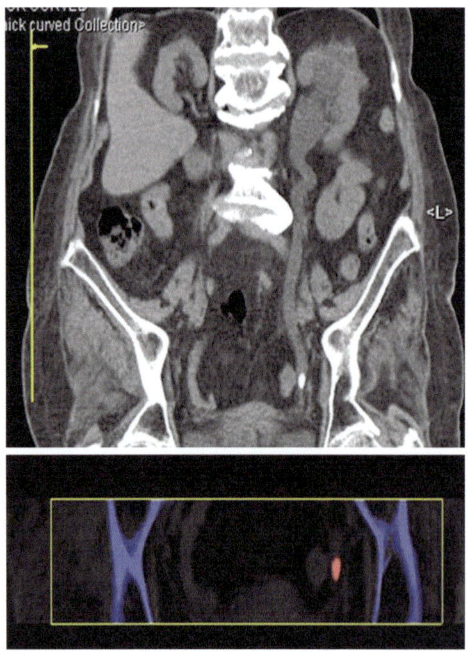

Fig. 5.10 Left ureteral stone in a patient with left acute flank pain. **a** Low-dose single-energy coronally reformatted CT image shows moderate left hydronephrosis due to an oval stone in the left pelvic ureter. **b** Dual-energy coronally reformatted CT image, obtained by using Kidney Stone software (Siemens Healthcare) with a "stone-targeted" protocol (scanning length 5 cm), demonstrated the uric acid composition (*red color*) of the stone

To summarize, in the clinical setting of kidney stone characterization, a CT protocol should consist of a combined low-dose single-energy CT acquisition of the whole urinary system completed with a dual-energy acquisition targeted to the anatomic region containing the stone. Uric acid stone can be identified by using dual-energy CT and correctly differentiated from calcified stone. Currently, owing to dual-energy spectra overlap, a definitive diagnosis cannot be posed for other stone types such as cystine and struvite.

References

1. Moe OW (2006) Kidney stones: pathophysiology and medical management. Lancet 367:333–344
2. Curhan GC (2007) Epidemiology of stone disease. Urol Clin North Am 34:287–293
3. Stamatelou KK, Francis ME, Jones CA et al (1994) Time trends in reported prevalence of kidney stones in the United States: 1976–1994. Kidney Int 63:1817–1823
4. Pak CY (1998) Kidney stones. Lancet 351: 1797–1801
5. Clark JY, Thompson IM, Optenberg SA (1995) Economic impact of urolithiasis in the United States. J Urol 154:2020–2024
6. Trinchieri A (2006) Epidemiological trends in urolithiasis: impact on our health care systems. Urol Res 34:151–156
7. Pollack HM (1990) Uroradiology. In: Pollack HM (ed) Clinical urography: an atlas and textbook of urological imaging, 3rd ed. Saunders, Philadelphia, pp 195–196
8. Sutherland JW, Parks JH, Coe FL (1985) Recurrence after a single renal stone in a community practice. Miner Electrolyte Metab 11:267–269
9. Daudon M, Donsimoni R, Hennequin C et al (2005) Sex- and age-related composition of 10 617 calculi analyzed by infrared spectroscopy. Urol Res 23:319–326
10. Smith RC, Verga M, McCarthy S et al (1996) Diagnosis of acute flank pain: value of unenhanced helical CT. AJR Am J Roentgenol 166:97–101
11. Smith RC, Varanelli M (2000) Diagnosis and management of acute ureterolithiasis: CT is truth. AJR Am J Roentgenol 175:3–6
12. Kambadakone AR, Eisner BH, Catalano OA et al (2010) New and evolving concepts in the imaging and management of urolithiasis: urologists' perspective. Radiographics 30:603–623
13. Bellin MF, Renard-Penna R, Conort P et al (2004) Helical CT evaluation of the chemical composition of urinary tract calculi with a discriminant analysis of CT-attenuation values and density. Eur Radiol 14:2134–2140
14. Miller OF, Rineer SK, Reicherd SR et al (1998) Prospective comparison of unenhanced helical computed tomography and intravenous urography in the evaluation of acute flank pain. Urology 52:982–987
15. Boulay I, Holtz P, Foley WD et al (1999) Ureteral calculi: diagnostic efficacy of helical CT and implications for treatment of patients. AJR Am J Roentgenol 172:1485–1490
16. Sourtzis S, Thibeau JF, Damry N et al (1999) Radiologic investigation of renal colic: unenhanced helical CT compared with excretory urography. AJR Am J Roentgenol 172:1491–1494
17. Preminger GM, Vieweg J, Leder RA et al (1998) Urolithiasis: detection and management with unenhanced spiral CT—a urologic perspective. Radiology 207:308–309
18. Smith RC, Rosenfield AT, Choe KA et al (1995) Acute flank pain: comparison of non-contrast-enhanced CT and intravenous urography. Radiology 194:789–794
19. Fielding JR, Silverman SG, Samuel S et al (1998) Unenhanced helical CT of ureteral stones: a replacement for excretory urography in planning treatment. AJR Am J Roentgenol 171:1051–1053
20. Fielding JR, Fox LA, Heller H et al (1997) Spiral CT in the evaluation of flank pain: overall accuracy and feature analysis. J Comput Assist Tomogr 21:635–638
21. Katz DS, Lane MJ, Sommer FG (1996) Unenhanced helical CT of ureteral stones: incidence of associated urinary tract findings. AJR Am J Roentgenol 166:1319–1322
22. Hamm M, Wawroschek F, Weckermann D et al (2001) Unenhanced helical computed tomography in the evaluation of acute flank pain. Eur Urol 39:460–465
23. Lin WC, Uppot RN, Li CS et al (2007) Value of automated coronal reformations from 64-section multidetector row computerized tomography in the diagnosis of urinary stone disease. J Urol 178:907–911
24. Dretler SP, Spencer BA (2001) CT and stone fragility. J Endourol 15:31–36
25. Saw KC, McAteer JA, Monga AG et al (2000) Helical CT of urinary calculi: effect of stone composition, stone size, and scan collimation. AJR Am J Roentgenol 175:329–332
26. Bruce RG, Munch LC, Hoven AD et al (1997) Urolithiasis associated with the protease inhibitor indinavir. Urology 50:513–518
27. Ege G, Akman H, Kuzucu K et al (2003) Acute ureterolithiasis: incidence of secondary signs on unenhanced helical CT and influence on patient management. Clin Radiol 58:990–994
28. Kawashima A, Sandler CM, Boridy IC et al (1997) Unenhanced helical CT of ureterolithiasis: value of the tissue rim sign. AJR Am J Roentgenol 168: 997–1000

29. Spielmann AL, Heneghan JP, Lee LJ et al (2002) Decreasing the radiation dose for renal stone CT: a feasibility study of single- and multidetector CT. AJR Am J Roentgenol 178:1058–1062
30. Brenner DJ, Hall EJ (2007) Computed tomography: an increasing source of radiation exposure. N Engl J Med 357:2277–2284
31. Tack D, Sourtzis S, Delpierre I et al (2003) Low-dose unenhanced multidetector CT of patients with suspected renal colic. AJR Am J Roentgenol 180:305–311
32. Ciaschini MW, Remer EM, Baker ME et al (2009) Urinary calculi: radiation dose reduction of 50% and 75% at CT—effect on sensitivity. Radiology 251:105–111
33. Denton ER, Mackenzie A, Greenwell T et al (1999) Unenhanced helical CT for renal colic: is the radiation dose justifiable? Clin Radiol 54:444–447
34. Mulkens TH, Daineffe S, De Wijngaert R et al (2007) Urinary stone disease: comparison of standard- dose and low-dose with 4D MDCT tube current modulation. AJR Am J Roentgenol 188:553–562
35. Hamm M, Knopfle E, Wartenberg S et al (2002) Low dose unenhanced helical computerized tomography for the evaluation of acute flank pain. J Urol 167:1687–1691
36. Kalra MK, Maher MM, Toth TL et al (2004) Techniques and applications of automatic tube current modulation for CT. Radiology 233:649–657
37. Funama Y, Awai K, Nakayama Y et al (2005) Radiation dose reduction without degradation of low-contrast detectability at abdominal multisection CT with a low-tube voltage technique: phantom study. Radiology 237:905–910
38. Schindera ST, Diedrichsen L, Muller HC et al (2011) Iterative reconstruction algorithm for abdominal multidetector CT at different tube voltages: assessment of diagnostic accuracy, image quality, and radiation dose in a phantom study. Radiology 260:454–462
39. Singh S, Kalra MK, Hsieh J et al (2010) Abdominal CT: comparison of adaptive statistical iterative and filtered back projection reconstruction techniques. Radiology 257:373–383
40. Sheir KZ, Mansour O, Madbouly K, Elsobky E et al (2005) Determination of the chemical composition of urinary calculi by noncontrast spiral computerized tomography. Urol Res 33:99–104
41. Deveci S, Cokun M, Tekin MI et al (2004) Spiral computed tomography: role in determination of chemical compositions of pure and mixed urinary stones—an in vitro study. Urology 64:237–240
42. Thomas C, Patschan O, Ketelsen D et al (2009) Dual-energy CT for the characterization of urinary calculi: In vitro and in vivo evaluation of a low-dose scanning protocol. Eur Radiol 19:1553–1559
43. Mostafavi MR, Ernst RD, Saltzman B (1998) Accurate determination of chemical composition of urinary calculi by spiral computerized tomography. J Urol 159:673–675
44. Sheir KZ, Mansour O, Madbouly K et al (2005) Determination of the chemical composition of urinary calculi by noncontrast spiral computerized tomography. Urol Res 33:99–104
45. Motley G, Dalrymple N, Keesling C et al (2001) Hounsfield unit density in the determination of urinary stone composition. Urology 58:170–173
46. Mitcheson HD, Zamenhof RG, Bankoff MS et al (1983) Determination of the chemical composition of urinary calculi by computerized tomography. J Urol 130:814–819
47. Stolzmann P, Leschka S, Scheffel H et al (2010) Characterization of urinary stones with dual-energy CT: improved differentiation using a tin filter. Invest Radiol 45:1–6
48. Qu M, Ramirez-Giraldo JC, Leng S et al (2011) Dual-Energy Dual-Source CT With Additional Spectral Filtration Can Improve the Differentiation of Non–Uric Acid Renal Stones: An Ex Vivo Phantom Study. AJR Am J Roentgenol 196:1279–1287
49. Qu M, Jaramillo-Alvarez G, Ramirez-Giraldo JC et al (2013) Urinary stone differentiation in patients with large body size using dual-energy dual-source computed tomography. Eur Radiol 23:1408–1414
50. Zilberman DE, Ferrandino MN, Preminger GM et al (2010) In vivo determination of urinary stone composition using dual energy computerized tomography with advanced post-acquisition processing. J Urol 184:2354–2359
51. Flohr TG, McCollough CH, Bruder H et al (2006) First performance evaluation of a dual-source CT (DSCT) system. Eur Radiol 16:256–268
52. Johnson TR, Krauss B, Sedlmair M et al (2007) Material differentiation by dual energy CT: initial experience. Eur Radiol 17:1510–1517
53. Primak AN, Fletcher JG, Vrtiska TJ et al (2007) Noninvasive differentiation of uric acid versus non-uric acid kidney stones using dual-energy CT. Acad Radiol 14:1441–1447
54. Stolzmann P, Kozomara M, Chuck N et al (2010) In vivo identification of uric acid stones with dual-energy CT: diagnostic performance evaluation in patients. Abdom Imaging 35:629–635
55. Matlaga BR, Kawamoto S, Fishman E (2008) Dual source computed tomography: a novel technique to determine stone composition. Urology 72:1164–1168
56. Boll DT, Patil NA, Paulson EK et al (2009) Renal stone assessment with dual-energy multidetector CT and advanced postprocessing techniques: improved characterization of renal stone composition—pilot study. Radiology 250:813–820
57. Hartman R, Kawashima A, Takahashi N et al (2012) Applications of dual- energy CT in urologic imaging: an update. Radiol Clin N Am 50:191–205
58. Kaza RK, Platt JF, Megibow AJ (2013) Dual-energy CT of the urinary tract. Abdom Imaging 38:167–179
59. Graser A, Johnson TR, Bader M et al (2008) Dual energy CT characterization of urinary calculi: initial in vitro and clinical experience. Invest Radiol 43: 112–119

60. Grosjean R, Sauer B, Guerra RM et al (2008) Characterization of human renal stones with MDCT: advantage of dual energy and limitations due to respiratory motion. AJR Am J Roentgenol 190: 720–728
61. Stolzmann P, Scheffel H, Rentsch K et al (2008) Dual-energy computed tomography for the differentiation of uric acid stones: ex vivo performance evaluation. Urol Res 36:133–138
62. Kulkarni NM, Eisner BH, Pinho DF et al (2013) Determination of renal stone composition in phantom and patients using single-source dual-energy computed tomography. J Comput Assist Tomogr 37:37–45
63. Duan X, Qu M, Wang J, et al (2012) Differentiation of calcium oxalate monohydrate and calcium oxalate dihydrate stones using quantitative morphological information from micro-computerized tomography and clinical computerized tomography images. J Urol. Doi:pii: S0022-5347(12)05469-9. 10.1016/j.juro.2012.11.004
64. Krauss B (2011) Dual Source CT (section 2.3). In: Johnson TRC et al (eds) Dual energy CT in clinical practice. Springer, Berlin Heidelberg, p 17
65. Primak AN (2011) Kidney Stones (section 2). In: Johnson TRC et al (eds) Dual energy CT in clinical practice. Springer, Berlin Heidelberg, p 17
66. Primak AN, Giraldo JC, Eusemann CD et al (2010) Dual-source dual-energy CT with additional tin filtration: Dose and image quality evaluation in phantoms and in vivo. AJR Am J Roentgenol 195:1164–1174
67. Primak AN, Ramirez Giraldo JC, Liu X et al (2009) Improved dual-energy material discrimination for dual-source CT by means of additional spectral filtration. Med Phys 36:1359–1369
68. Manglaviti G, Tresoldi S, Guerrer CS et al (2011) In vivo evaluation of the chemical composition of urinary stones using dual-energy CT. AJR Am J Roentgenol 197:W76–W83
69. Jepperson MA, Thiel DD, Cernigliaro JG et al (2012) Determination of ureter stent appearance on dual-energy computed tomography scan. Urology 80: 986–989
70. Li XH, Zhao R, Liu B et al (2013) Determination of urinary stone composition using dual-energy spectral CT: Initial in vitro analysis. Clin Radiol. doi:pii: S0009-9260(13)00073-1
71. Hidas G, Eliahou R, Duvdevani M et al (2010) Determination of renal stone composition with dual-energy CT: in vivo analysis and comparison with x-ray diffraction. Radiology 257:394–401
72. Ascenti G, Siragusa C, Racchiusa S et al (2010) Stone-targeted dual-energy CT: a new diagnostic approach to urinary calculosis. AJR Am J Roentgenol 195:953–958

6 Adrenal Glands

Achille Mileto, Daniele Marin, Lisa M. Ho and Rendon C. Nelson

6.1 Introduction

The adrenal glands can develop a myriad of abnormalities, which can be fundamentally differentiated into benign or malignant lesions having either hyperfunction or non-hyperfunction (i.e., non-function) [1, 2]. Functioning lesions typically secrete hormonal metabolites and include a variety of tumors, some of which are very rare. These tumors can produce cortisol, aldosterone, and sex hormones as well as adrenergic hormones in the case of pheochromocytomas [1–3]. Non-functioning tumors are far more common and include both benign and malignant lesions. Benign masses include cortical adenomas, myelolipomas, cysts and less commonly ganglioneuromas, hemangioendotheliomas, hemorrhage, and granulomatous disease. Malignant lesions include metastases, lymphoma, neuroblastoma, adrenocortical carcinoma, and some forms of pheochromocytomas [1–3].

Before the advent of cross-sectional imaging, many adrenal lesions remained undiagnosed and were only found at autopsy [4–7]. The widespread use of CT and MR has led to increased detection of adrenal lesions, many of which are incidentally detected during imaging for unrelated reasons. This emphasizes the importance of accurate adrenal lesion characterization by imaging [7–11].

Adrenal gland abnormalities are observed in up to 5–8 % of patients undergoing CT, with a high incidence of lesions in older patients [12]. Most of these masses are benign, whereas the others are usually adrenal metastases [13, 14]. The prevalence of adrenal metastases in patients with extra-adrenal cancer, most frequently from lung and kidney carcinomas, ranges between 32 and 73 % in different series [1, 12].

The characterization of adrenal lesions in patients with a known extra-adrenal primary carcinoma has a major clinical importance. For example, an isolated ipsilateral adrenal metastasis in a patient with resectable primary non-small cell lung cancer is treated as localized disease. In these patients (about 9 %), resection of an isolated adrenal metastasis has been shown to extend disease-free survival [7–10, 14]. Therefore, the main diagnostic challenge is differentiating between benign adenomas and adrenal metastases.

6.2 State of the Art Conventional (Multi-detector) CT

It is well-established that determining the presence of microscopic intracellular lipid content with unenhanced CT is a very accurate way to differentiate benign adenomas from non-adenomatous lesions [6, 12]. This finding is based on the consolidated evidence that up to 70 % of adrenal adenomas contain abundant intracellular fat (mainly cholesterol, fatty acids, and neutral fat), whereas almost all malignant lesions do not [12, 15–20]. Lee et al. [6] first

G. Ascenti et al., *CT of the Retroperitoneum*,
DOI: 10.1007/978-88-470-5469-1_6, © Springer-Verlag Italia 2014

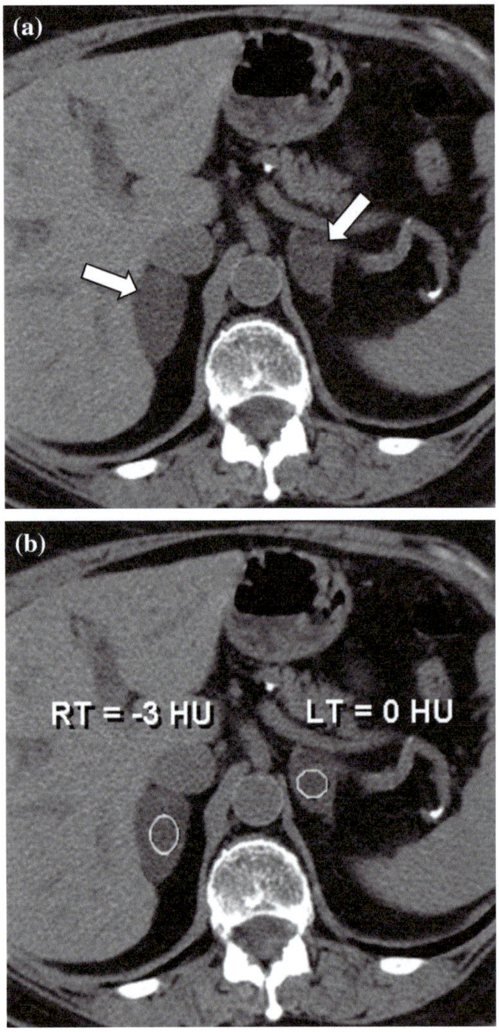

Fig. 6.1 Example of the unenhanced CT densitometry technique in lipid-rich adrenal adenomas. Unenhanced image (**a**) shows incidental lesions (*arrows*) in both adrenal glands. ROIs placed within both lesions (**b**) reveals an attenuation of −3 and 0 HU, respectively, consistent with adenomas

demonstrated that there is an inverse linear relationship between intracellular fat content and attenuation on unenhanced CT.

The CT densitometry technique involves placement of a region-of-interest (ROI) over one-half to two-thirds of the lesion surface area, avoiding necrotic or hemorrhagic regions [12]. The measurement should be made on a CT section acquired through the center of the lesion to avoid partial-volume effects from adjacent retroperitoneal fat (Fig. 6.1). The +10-HU threshold is used as a standard reference point from which lipid-rich adrenal adenomas can be differentiated from non-adenomatous lesions on unenhanced CT scans. If the lesion has an attenuation less than or equal to +10 HU, it can be considered benign, with a sensitivity of 71 % and specificity of 98 % [2, 3, 7, 12].

Although the detection of intracellular lipid content is a sensitive and specific finding, many adrenal lesions have an attenuation value greater than +10 HU on unenhanced CT scans, as do almost all malignant lesions (Fig. 6.2). Therefore, these lesions are considered indeterminate, and other tests are generally required for further characterization [2, 3, 7, 12, 21–23].

Some authors have suggested that the CT densitometry technique can be improved if a histogram analysis of the distribution of attenuation numbers is used [12, 24]. Bae et al. [24] found the histogram method to be far more sensitive than the +10-HU threshold method in characterizing adrenal lesions on unenhanced images. This method also involves placement of an ROI over approximately one-half to two-thirds of the adrenal lesion surface area. This ROI is then post-processed with a histogram analysis tool that permits calculation of the number and range of pixel attenuation measurements (Fig. 6.3) [12, 24]. Recent studies proposed the use of a 10 % threshold to improve the accuracy of this technique to characterize some adenomas that would otherwise be considered indeterminate by mean CT attenuation alone (Figs. 6.4, 6.5) [25, 26]. A more recent study found that the combination of 18-FDG PET/CT with standard uptake values (SUV) and CT histogram analysis further improves the diagnostic accuracy of adrenal lesions characterization, yielding a sensitivity of 100 % and specificity of 97.3 % [27].

Secondary imaging findings that suggest an adrenal lesion has a benign nature include lesion size (most adenomas tend to measure less than 3 cm), smooth margins and uniform shape [2, 3, 7, 12, 21–23, 28, 29].

Up to 30 % of adenomas contain only small amounts of intracellular lipids (so-called "*lipid-poor adenomas*") and cannot be characterized

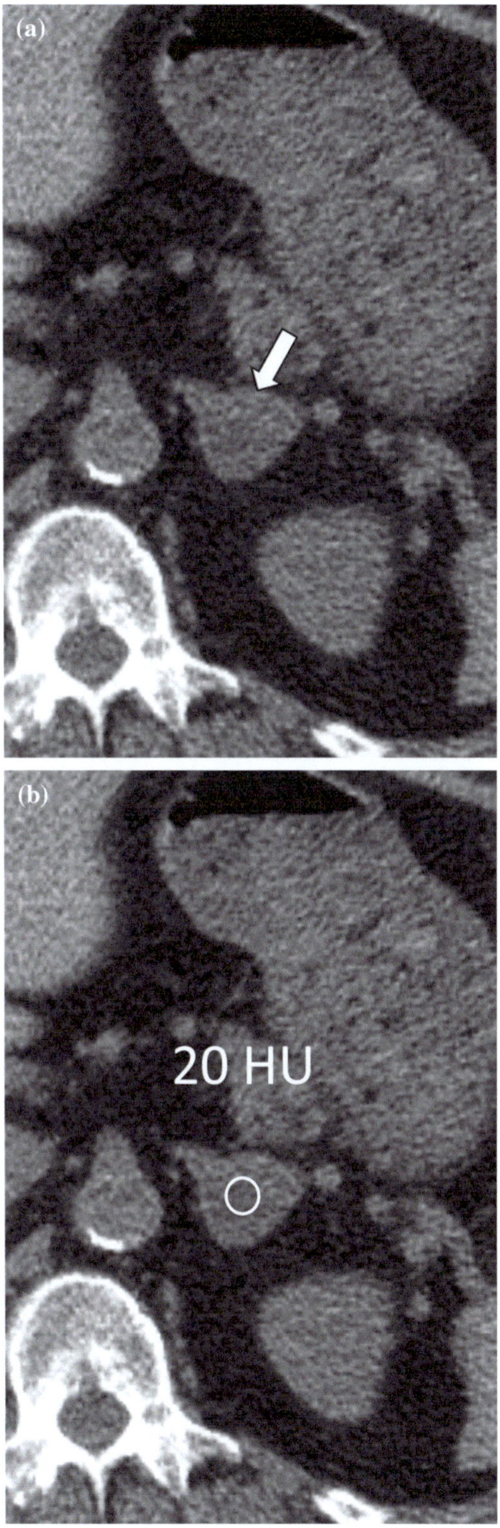

Fig. 6.2 Example of the unenhanced CT densitometry technique in lipid-poor adrenal adenoma. Unenhanced image (**a**) shows an incidental lesion (*arrow*) in the left adrenal gland. ROI measurement (**b**) shows an attenuation value greater than +10 HU. Therefore, this lesion is considered indeterminate, and other tests are required to characterize it

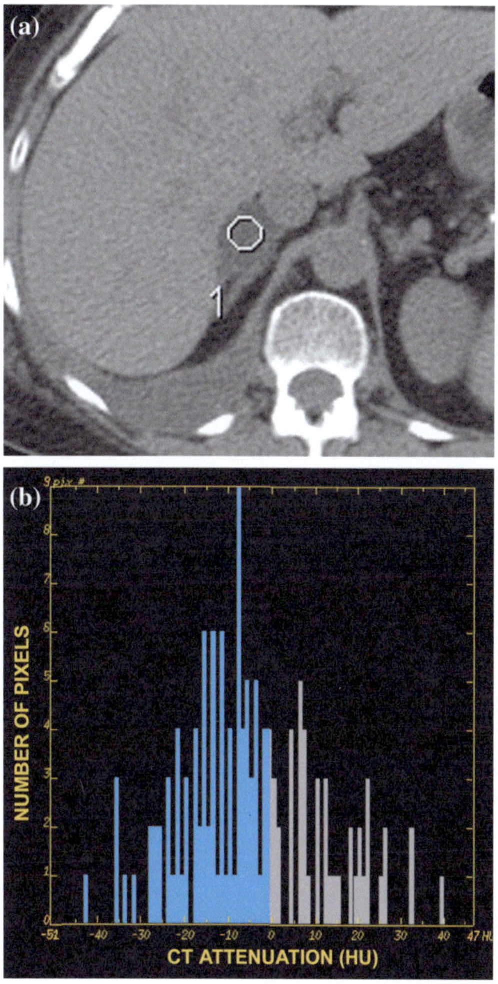

Fig. 6.3 Example of CT histogram analysis in a lipid-rich adrenal adenoma. An ROI is placed within the lesion on an unenhanced image (**a**). The ROI is then post-processed with a histogram analysis (**b**) measuring the number and range of pixel attenuation measurements within the lesion. The total number of examined pixels is 135, of which 92 (68 %) have an attenuation measuring less than 0 HU

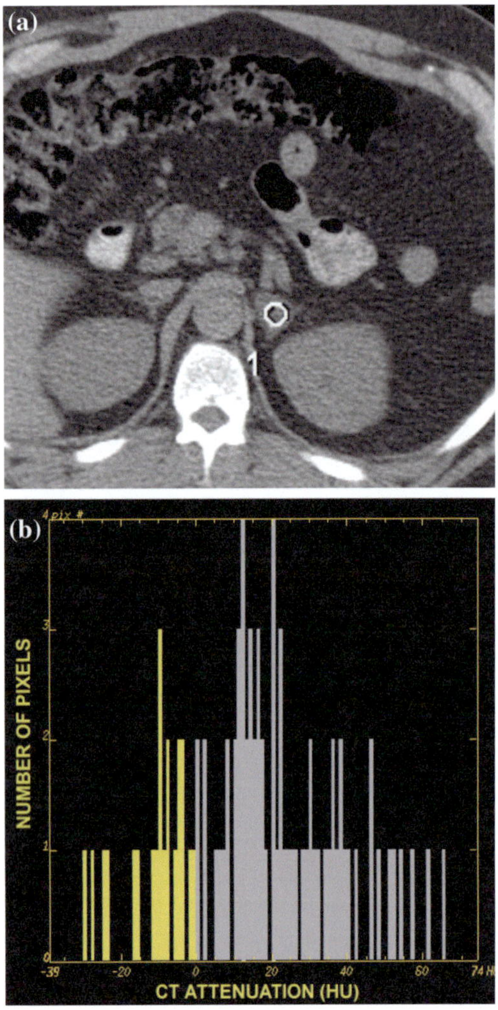

Fig. 6.4 Example of CT histogram analysis in a lipid-poor adrenal adenoma. An ROI is placed within the lesion on the unenhanced image (**a**). The ROI is then post-processed with a histogram analysis (**b**) measuring the number and range of pixel attenuation measurements within the lesion. The total number of examined pixels is 89, of which 20 (22 %) have an attenuation measuring less than 0 HU

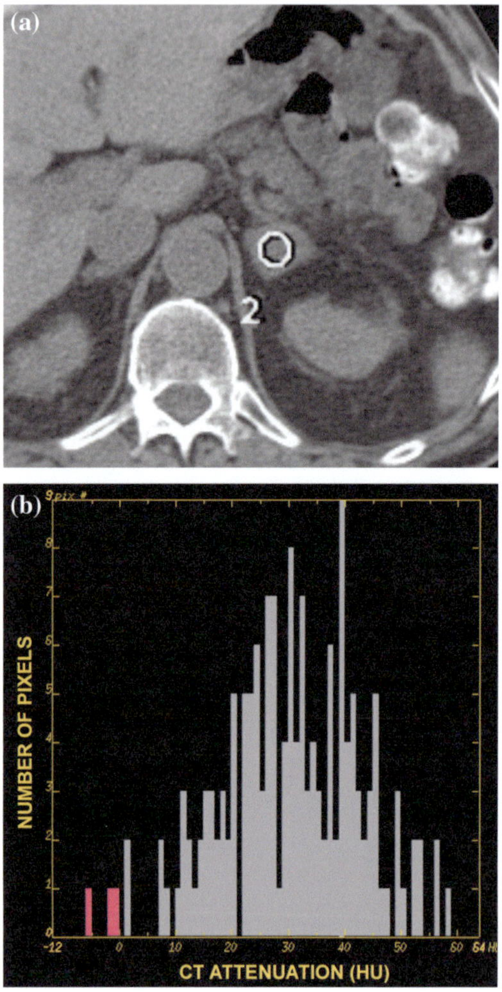

Fig. 6.5 Example of CT histogram analysis in an adrenal metastasis. An ROI is placed within the lesion on the unenhanced image (**a**). The ROI is then post-processed with a histogram analysis (**b**) measuring the number and range of pixel attenuation measurements within the lesion. The total number of examined pixels is 156, 3 of which (2 %) have an attenuation measuring less than 0 HU

with unenhanced CT densitometry techniques. Additional workup with contrast-enhanced CT or MRI is thus necessary to diagnose such challenging lesions [21–23, 28, 29]. The use of contrast-enhanced CT as an accurate technique for distinguishing between adrenal adenomas and non-adenomatous lesions was first described in the late 1990s. Boland et al., [30] first demonstrated that non-adenomatous adrenal lesions have significantly higher attenuation than adenomas on delayed CT scans obtained at arbitrarily chosen times (between 6 and 30 min) after the administration of contrast media. In particular, it was noticed that intravenous contrast media tended to "washout" much faster, sometimes as early as 3 min, from adenomatous lesions compared with non-adenomatous lesions and that the CT attenuation values began to approximate the unenhanced values [12]. Initially, one absolute CT attenuation measurement on a delayed scan was proposed [12, 31]. However, since delayed CT measurements depend on several factors (i.e., type, total dose, and injection rate of intravenous contrast media as well as the cardiac output of the patient), evidence in the literature failed to reproduce high accuracy when attempting to characterize adrenal lesion using an absolute attenuation measurement [8, 12, 32]. It was observed, however, that the ratio of adrenal attenuation measurements on the washout-delayed scan to the attenuation on the initial dynamic enhanced scan (during the portal venous phase using a 70 s delay) could characterize adrenal lesions with greater precision (Figs. 6.6, 6.7, 6.8) [12, 29]. Korobkin et al. [28] described a threshold enhancement washout value of 40 % for the diagnosis of adrenal adenomas, which yielded a sensitivity of 96 % and specificity of 100 %. The *relative percentage washout* is calculated by dividing the difference in attenuation (HU) between the portal venous and delayed phases by the attenuation (HU) during the portal venous phase, multiplied by 100 [12, 29]. If an unenhanced scan has been obtained, an *absolute percentage washout* can be calculated by dividing the difference in attenuation (HU) between the portal venous and delayed phases by the difference in attenuation (HU) between the portal venous and unenhanced phases, multiplied by 100 (Fig. 6.9). Based on the evidence from several studies [12, 29, 30, 33, 34], both *absolute and relative percentage washout* calculations are reliable, reproducible, and accurate methods for distinguishing adenomatous from non-adenomatous adrenal lesions in daily clinical practice. Although some debate still persists over the optimal threshold value, most authorities agree that, using a 15 min delayed scan, the optimal threshold values are 60 and 40 % for the *absolute and relative percentage washout*, respectively [2, 3, 7, 12, 21, 23].

Although the validity of these thresholds by using 15- or 10-minute delayed enhancement acquisition has been demonstrated [19, 29, 30, 33, 34], for efficiency reasons a protocol with a shorter time delay would be desirable. In fact, in some patients, delayed scans cannot be obtained because of the need to modify the CT schedule, and imaging directed at the adrenal glands may thus require a return visit to the radiology department, with additional exposure to radiation and contrast media thereby increasing the cost. A recent study by Kamiyama, et al. [35] demonstrated that the use of a 5-minute delayed CT acquisition can yield a high diagnostic accuracy in the differentiation of adenomatous from non-adenomatous adrenal lesions that is comparable with the accuracy for previous studies which used longer delay times ranging from 15 to 60 min [29, 30, 33, 34]. However, there continue to be concerns that a scan delay shorter than 15 min is not an enough washout time to allow for reliable separation between adenomas and non-adenomas. This is in part due to a recent study by Sangwaiya et al. [36] who refuted results from a previous publication [29] by demonstrating that the washout on a 10-min delayed scan had reduced sensitivity for the characterization of adrenal adenomas [36].

Overall, according to Boland et al. [12], when an adrenal lesion is encountered, it is helpful to employ a diagnostic algorithm for the use of multi-detector CT (MDCT) (Fig. 6.10) [3, 12, 19, 21–23]. The radiologist has to consider the following two points: (1) the age of the patient (metastases are less common in younger patients) and (2) the hormonal tests (to rule-out a hyperfunctioning tumor). The next two steps to be addressed are as follows: (3) whether the patient has a history of malignancy and (4) the availability of prior imaging examinations through the adrenal glands (e.g., a lumbar spine CT scan). If a lesion is stable on serial imaging for at least 6 months, the lesion can confidently assumed to be benign; on the other hand, significant growth, particularly in a patient with an underlying malignancy, strongly suggests metastatic disease [21–23]. If no prior imaging is available, unenhanced CT is required. Those lesions $\leq +10$ HU are deemed lipid-rich and benign. If the CT attenuation is $\geq +10$ HU, a dynamic and delayed contrast-enhanced CT for

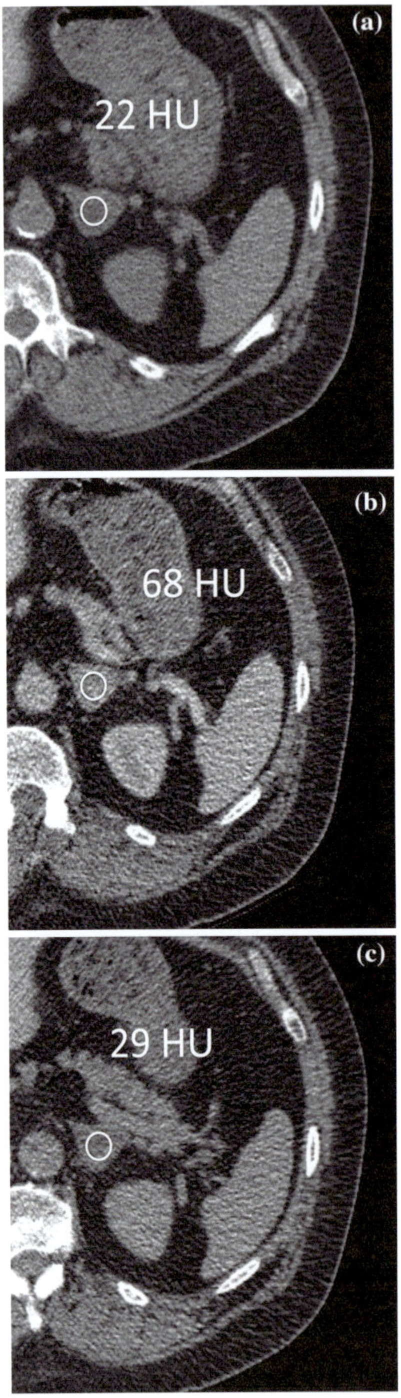

Fig. 6.6 Example of a washout % calculation in a lipid-poor adrenal adenoma. Based on unenhanced (**a**), contrast-enhanced portal venous (**b**) and delayed (**c**) phase attenuation values, the lesion demonstrated absolute washout of 85 % (39/46 × 100) and was characterized as an adenoma

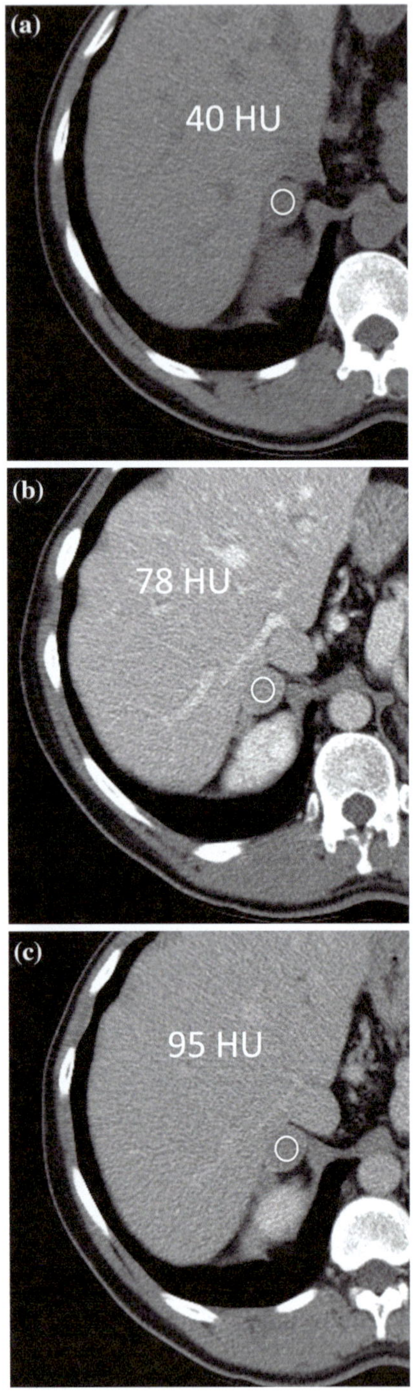

Fig. 6.7 Example of a washout % calculation in an adrenal metastasis from non-small cell lung cancer. Based on unenhanced (**a**), contrast-enhanced portal venous (**b**) and delayed (**c**) phase attenuation values, the lesion showed absolute washout of 45 % (17/38 × 100) and was characterized as a metastasis

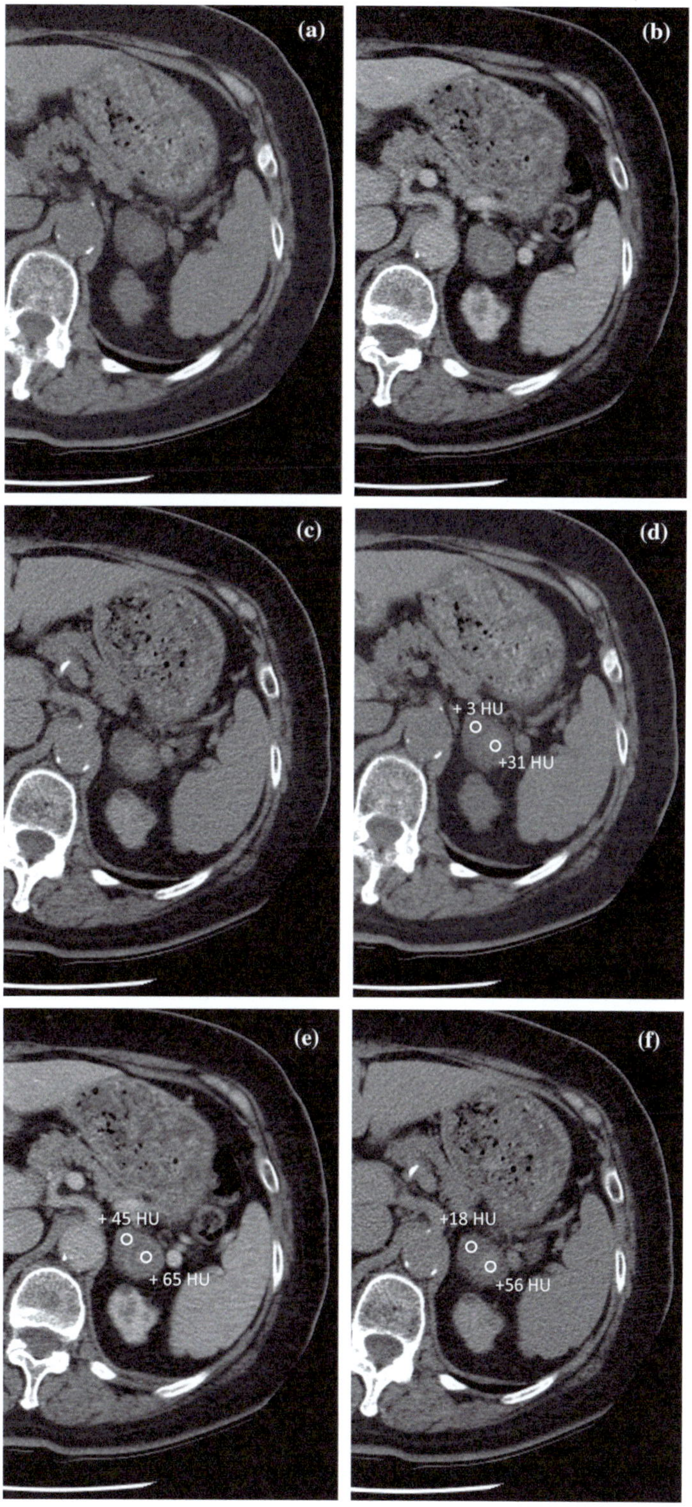

Fig. 6.8 Example of a washout % calculation in an adrenal collision tumor consisting of an adenoma and metastasis from non-small cell lung cancer. The lesion visually shows two different components, anteriorly and posteriorly, on unenhanced (**a**), contrast-enhanced portal venous (**b**) and delayed (**c**) phase images. Based on unenhanced (**d**), contrast-enhanced portal venous (**e**) and delayed (**f**) phase attenuation values, the anterior component demonstrated absolute washout of 64 % (27/42 × 100) and is characterized as an adenoma, The posterior component demonstrated absolute washout of 26 % (9/34 x 100) and is characterized as a metastasis

Wash-out %	***Equation***	***Wash-out % thresholds***	
		Adenoma	Nonadenoma
Absolute wash-out %	(Enhanced attenuation value –Delayed attenuation value) / (Enhanced attenuation value –Unenhanced attenuation value) X 100	> 60	< 60
Relative wash-out %	(Enhanced attenuation value –Delayed attenuation value) / Enhanced attenuation value X 100	> 40	< 40

Fig. 6.9 Summary of absolute and relative washout % calculation

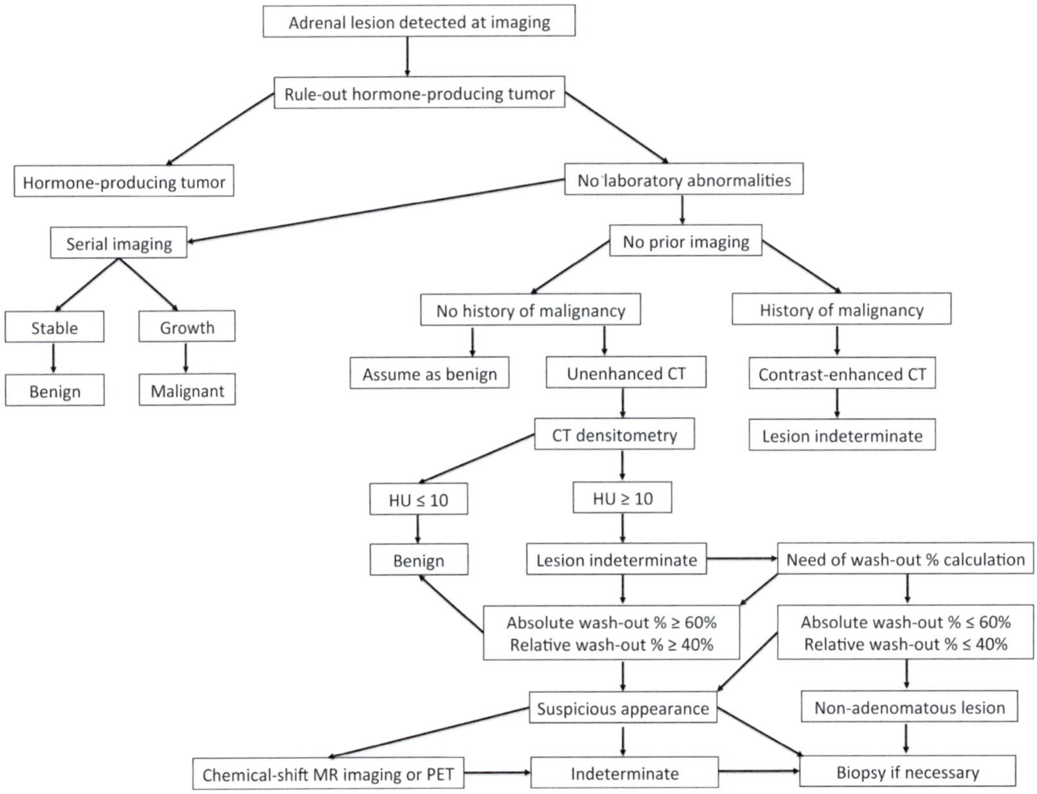

Fig. 6.10 MDCT diagnostic algorithm for incidental adrenal lesion [23]

calculating the % washout is required. Most lesions at this point will be characterized adequately with no need for further testing. However, a small percentage of lesions may benefit from chemical-shift MRI or 18-FDG PET [2, 12]. If a lesion remain indeterminate after these additional examinations, percutaneous biopsy may be considered. Alternatively, for young patients with no history of malignancy, a 6-month interval follow-up CT may be considered [21–23].

A diagnostic dilemma that is encountered on a frequent basis is the discovery of an incidental adrenal nodule on abdominal and chest CT scans performed for other reasons. In most of these patients, delayed imaging through the adrenal glands is not available. On contrast-enhanced CT scans acquired during either the arterial of venous phases, adrenal lesions enhance in an unpredictable fashion, thereby precluding the determination of a useful and reproducible attenuation threshold [2, 12, 21–23]. Thus, characterization of an incidental adrenal mass as either benign or malignant is not possible on single-phase contrast-enhanced CT. A dedicated adrenal CT protocol consists of unenhanced and contrast-enhanced early and delayed acquisitions. In practicality, when an incidental adrenal nodule is noted, many patients are rescheduled to be rescanned with a different CT protocol on a different day. Some of these patients will be directed toward another modality such MRI or PET.

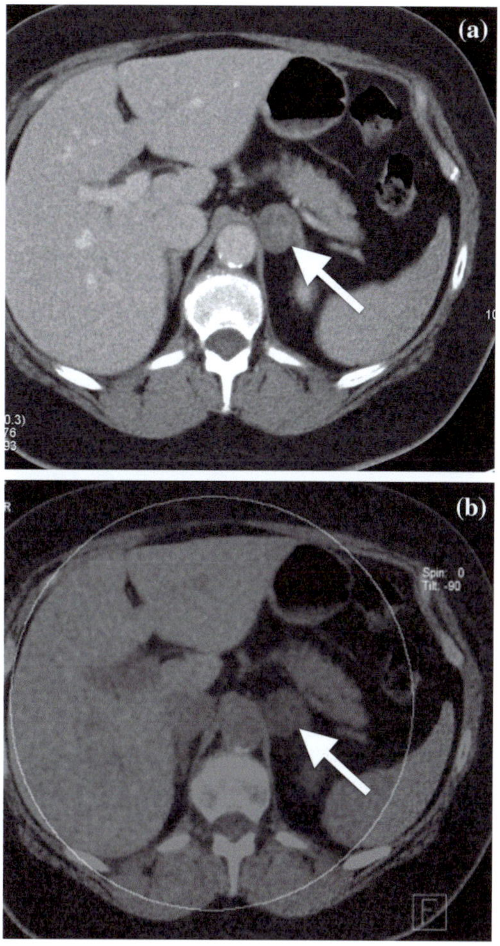

Fig. 6.11 Example of dual-energy, dual-source CT workflow in a left adrenal adenoma. An incidental lesion (arrow) is visible on portal venous phase image (**a**). By means of iodine subtraction from a dual-energy contrast-enhanced dataset a virtual unenhanced image series (**b**) is created. Note the white ring which corresponds to the field-of-view on the tube with the smaller detector (26 cm)

6.3 Spectral CT: Study Protocols and Clinical Applications

Spectral CT has been shown to be an effective and reliable tool for accurately characterize adrenal lesions by means of dual-energy scanning.

Spectral CT assessment of adrenal lesions relies on two main assumptions. First, lipid-containing tissues undergo a characteristic decrease in attenuation as tube voltage is decreased due to the unique CT attenuation properties of fat at different tube voltage settings. Second, virtual-unenhanced images, reconstructed from contrast-enhanced dual-energy CT data with selective spectral-based iodine extraction, have been shown to have sufficient accuracy and may be able to replace standard unenhanced images (Fig. 6.11) [37, 38]. In actuality, however, results from some of the first studies on the appearance of adrenal adenomas at low (e.g., 80 kVp) and high (e.g., 140 kVp) energies had been mixed. In a preliminary investigation of the attenuation values of adrenal adenomas, Kalra et al. [39] reported a decrease in mean attenuation of 20 ± 5.5 HU (range, 0–38) at 80 kVp from that at 140 kVp (n = 17 adenomas in 16 patients). In another follow-up study of 69 adenomas in 58 patients imaged at 80 and 120 kVp, a decrease in mean attenuation of only 3.3 HU (range, 0–25 HU) was reported [40]. In a more recent study [37] of adrenal nodules using unenhanced dual-energy CT at 80 and 140 kVp, 13 (50 %) of 26 adenomas had a mean attenuation decrease in 0.4 ± 7.1 HU on the 80-kVp images relative to the 140 kVp images, indicative of the presence of intracellular lipid within an adenoma (Fig. 6.12). All 5 metastatic lesions demonstrated a relative increase in attenuation increase as the kVp was decrease from 80 to 140. Therefore, a measurable decrease in attenuation of an adrenal lesion on 80-kVp images relative to the attenuation of the lesion on the 140-kVp images is a highly specific sign of microscopic lipid in adrenal adenomas. However, the sensitivity of this technique is low because some adenomas, possibly lipid-poor adenomas, demonstrate an increase in attenuation at 80-kVp [37]. Some authors have speculated that this phenomenon could be related to the relative proportion of intracellular lipid and soft tissue within adenomas, unlike subcutaneous fat, which has a more uniform fat content and attenuation [37].

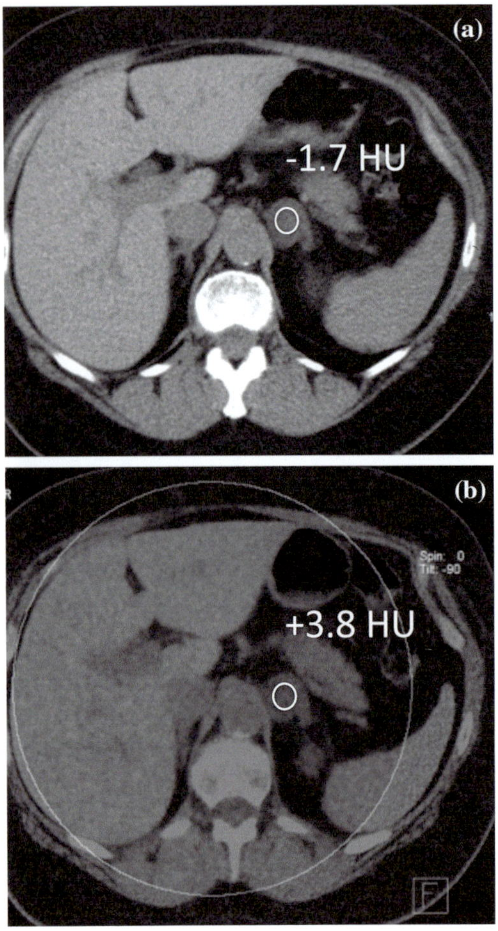

Fig. 6.12 Standard true unenhanced image and virtual unenhanced image from a dual-energy dataset in a patient with a left adrenal adenoma. A substantial concordance of HU attenuation measurements between standard true unenhanced (**a**) and virtual unenhanced (**b**) images is shown. Note that the two image series can be easily discriminated, since virtual unenhanced images appears slightly more grainy than conventional unenhanced series due to the lower kVp and smoothing induced by the post-processing algorithm

In another study, Gnannt et al. [41] scanned 39 incidental adrenal nodules using contrast-enhanced dual-energy CT. In this study, virtual-unenhanced images were generated from the dual-energy series in an individualized fashion by replacing manufacturer default values for soft tissue and fat attenuation with attenuation measurements of spleen and subcutaneous fat, respectively. In comparison with standard unenhanced images as a reference standard, the sensitivity, specificity, and accuracy in diagnosing lipid-rich adrenal adenomas with virtual enhanced images were 91–95, 100, and 95–97 %, respectively [41].

Recently, Ho et al. [42] confirmed that virtual non-contrast attenuation measurements of adrenal nodules have high concordance with true non-contrast attenuation measurements (Fig. 6.13). These measurements are reproducible among radiologists with different levels of clinical experience. This study concluded that virtual non-contrast image reconstruction has the potential to replace true non-contrast imaging for the initial characterization of incidentally discovered adrenal nodules found on contrast-enhanced dual-energy CT [42].

More recently, a study by Kim et al. [43] showed that the attenuation values measured on virtual-unenhanced CT images tend to be higher than those measured on unenhanced images. In this study, virtual-unenhanced images were created by subtracting iodine from both early and delayed contrast-enhanced CT images. Many lipid-rich adenomas were not correctly diagnosed on virtual unenhanced CT and, as a result, these authors concluded that virtual-unenhanced CT images have lower sensitivity for lipid-rich adenoma than unenhanced CT. However, their adrenal protocol using dual-energy CT with virtual-unenhanced images had the same sensitivity for adenomas as the adrenal protocol CT with real unenhanced images. This finding is likely due to the improvement in performance that occurs with the analysis of washout is included in the protocol. In this

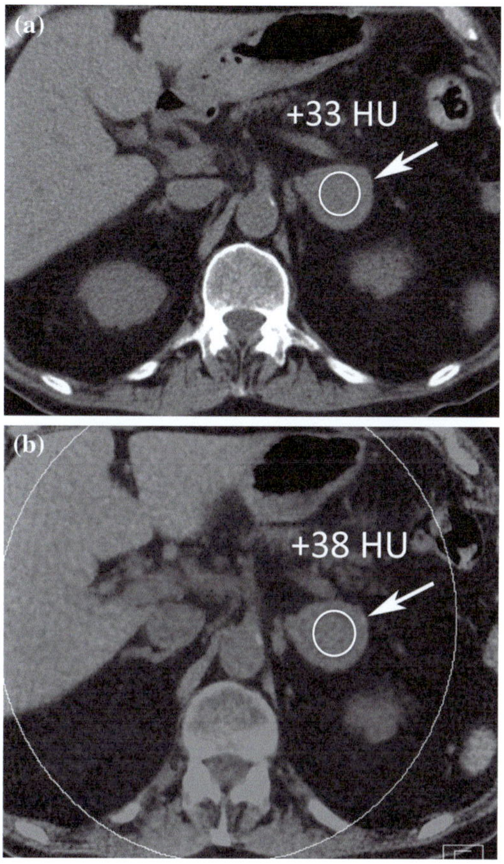

Fig. 6.13 Standard true unenhanced image and virtual-unenhanced image from a dual-energy dataset in a patient with a left adrenal metastasis. A substantial concordance of HU attenuation measurements between standard true unenhanced (**a**) and virtual unenhanced (**b**) images is shown

study, the potential omission of the true non-contrast acquisition resulted in a radiation saving of 27 % [43].

Overall, preliminary evidence suggest that both lipid-rich and lipid-poor adenomas may be characterized by means of spectral-based analysis with a sensitivity of 100 % when contrast media washout analysis is included. However, virtual-unenhanced images derived from iodine subtraction cannot accurately diagnose a substantial number of lipid-rich adenomas due to the technical failure of spectral-based iodine subtraction from the contrast-enhanced CT images. As a result, many of the patients with a lipid-rich adenoma would not be accurately diagnosed by using virtual-unenhanced CT alone, making it necessary to include a delayed scan to determine the washout characteristics.

With further technical improvements in iodine spectral subtraction, unenhanced CT may no longer be an essential component of the adrenal protocol CT when patients are imaged with dual-energy CT.

References

1. Young WF Jr (2007) The incidentally discovered adrenal mass. N Engl J Med 356:601–610
2. Boland GW, Blake MA, Hahn PF, Mayo-Smith WW (2008) Incidental adrenal lesions: principles, techniques, and algorithms for imaging characterization. Radiology 249:756–775
3. Boland GW (2011) Adrenal Imaging. Abdom Imaging 36:472–482
4. Song J, Chaudhry FS, Mayo-Smith WW (2008) The incidental adrenal mass on CT: prevalence of adrenal disease in 1,049 consecutive adrenal masses in patients with no known malignancy. AJR Am J Roentgenol 190:1163–1168
5. Dunnick NR, Korobkin M (2002) Imaging of adrenal incidentalomas. AJR Am J Roentgenol 179:559–568
6. Lee MJ, Hahn PF, Papanicolou N et al (1991) Benign and malignant adrenal masses: CT distinction with attenuation coefficients, size, and observer analysis. Radiology 179:415–418
7. Blake MA, Cronin CG, Boland GW (2010) Adrenal Imaging. AJR Am J Roentgenol 194:1450–1460
8. Dunnick NR, Korobkin M (2002) Imaging of adrenal incidentalomas: current status. AJR 179:559–568
9. Lam KY, Lo CY (2002) Metastatic tumours of the adrenal glands: a 30-year experience in a teaching hospital. Clin Endocrinol 56:95–101
10. Mitchell IC, Nwariaku FE (2007) Adrenal masses in the cancer patient: surveillance or excision. Oncologist 12:168–174
11. Bovio S, Cataldi A, Reimondo G et al (2006) Prevalence of adrenal incidentaloma in a contemporary computerized tomography series. J Endocrinol Invest 29:298–302
12. Boland GWL, Blake MA, Hahn PF, Mayo-Smith WW (2008) Incidental adrenal lesions: principles, techniques, and algorithms for imaging characterization. Radiology 249:756–775
13. Angeli A, Osella G, Ali A et al (1997) Adrenal incidentaloma: an overview of clinical and epidemiological data from the National Italian Study Group. Horm Res 47:279–283
14. Ettinghausen SE, Burt ME (1991) Prospective evaluation of unilateral adrenal masses in patients

with operable non-small-cell lung cancer. J Clin Oncol 9:1462–1466
15. Korobkin M, Giordano TJ, Brodeur FJ et al (1996) Adrenal adenomas: relationship between histologic lipid and CT and MR findings. Radiology 200:743–747
16. Anderson JB, Gray GF (1989) Adrenal pathology. In: Vaughan ED, Carey RM (eds) Adrenal disorders. Thieme Medical, New York, pp 18–19
17. Carney JA (1992) Adrenal gland. In: Sternberg SS (ed) Histology for pathologists. Raven, New York, pp 150–154
18. Lee MJ, Hahn PF, Papanicolau N et al (1991) Benign and malignant adrenal masses: CT distinction with attenuation coefficients, size, and observer analysis. Radiology 179:415–418
19. Caoili EM, Korobkin M, Francis IR et al (2002) Adrenal masses: characterization with combined unenhanced and delayed enhanced CT. Radiology 222:629–633
20. Hahn PF, Blake MA, Boland GW (2006) Adrenal lesions: attenuation measurement differences between CT scanners. Radiology 240:458–463
21. Boland GWL (2010) Adrenal Imaging: Why, When, What, and How? Part 1. Why and When to Image? AJR Am J Roentgenol 95:W377–W381
22. Boland GWL (2011) Adrenal imaging: why, when, what, and how? Part 2. Why and when to image? AJR Am J Roentgenol 196:W1–W5
23. Boland GWL (2011) Adrenal imaging: why, when, what, and how? Part 3. The algorithmic approach to definitive characterization of the adrenal incidentaloma. AJR Am J Roentgenol 196:W109–W111
24. Bae KT, Fuangtharnthip P, Prasad SR, Joe BN, Heiken JP (2003) Adrenal masses: CT characterization with histogram analysis method. Radiology 228:735–742
25. Remer EM, Motta-Ramirez GA, Shepardson LB, Hamrahian AH, Herts BR (2006) CT histogram analysis in pathologically proven adrenal masses. AJR Am J Roentgenol 187:191–196
26. Ho LM, Paulson EK, Brady MJ, Wong TZ, Schindera ST (2008) Lipid-Poor adenomas on unenhanced CT: does histogram analysis increase sensitivity compared with a mean attenuation threshold? AJR Am J Roentgenol 191:234–238
27. Perri M, Erba P, Volterrani D et al (2011) Adrenal masses in patients with cancer: PET/CT characterization with combined CT histogram and standardized uptake value PET analysis. AJR Am J Roentgenol 197:209–216
28. Korobkin M, Brodeur FJ, Francis IR, Quint LE, Dunnick NR, Londy F (1998) CT time-attenuation wash-out curves of adrenal adenomas and nonadenomas. AJR Am J Roentgenol 170:747–752
29. Szolar DH, Kammerhuber FH (1998) Adrenal adenomas and nonadenomas: assessment of wash-out at delayed contrast-enhanced CT. Radiology 207:369–375
30. Boland GW, Hahn PF, Pena C, Mueller PR (1997) Adrenal masses: characterization with delayed contrast-enhanced CT. Radiology 202:693–696
31. Kloos RT, Gross MD, Francis IR et al (1995) Incidentally discovered adrenal masses. Endocr Rev 16:460–484
32. Korobkin M (2000) CT characterization of adrenal masses: the time has come. Radiology 217:629–632
33. Pena CS, Boland GW, Hahn PF, Lee MJ, Mueller PR (2000) Characterization of indeterminate (lipid-poor) adrenal masses: use of washout characteristics at contrast-enhanced CT. Radiology 217:798–802
34. Blake MA, Kalra MK, Sweeney AT et al (2005) Distinguishing benign from malignant adrenal masses: multi-detector row CT protocol with 10-minute delay. Radiology 238:578–585
35. Kamiyama T, Fukukura Y, Yoneyama T, Takumi K, Nakajo M (2008) Distinguishing adrenal adenomas from nonadenomas: combined use of diagnostic parameters of unenhanced and short 5-minute dynamic enhanced CT protocol. Radiology 250: 474–481
36. Sangwaiya MJ, Boland GWL, Cronin CG, Blake MA, Halpern EF, Hahn PF (2010) Incidental adrenal lesions: accuracy of characterization with contrast-enhanced washout multidetector CT—10-minute delayed imaging protocol revisited in a large patient cohort. Radiology 256:504–510
37. Gupta RT, Ho LM, Marin D, Boll DT, Barnhart HX, Nelson RC (2010) Dual energy CT for characterization of adrenal nodules: initial experience. AJR Am J Roentgenol 194:1479–1483
38. Coursey CA, Nelson RC, Boll DT et al (2010) Dual-energy multidetector CT: how does it work, what can it tell us, and when can we use it in abdominopelvic imaging? Radiographics 30:1037–1055
39. Kalra M, Blake M, Sahani D, Hahn P, Mueller P, Boland G (2007) Dual energy CT for characterization of adrenal adenomas (abstr). In: Radiological Society of North America scientific assembly and annual meeting program. Oak Brook, Ill: Radiological Society of North America, 347
40. Boland G, Jagtiani M, Kambadakone Ramesh A, Hahn P, Sahani D, Kalra M (2008) Characterization of lipid poor adrenal adenomas: accuracy of dual energy CT (abstr). In: Radiological Society of North America scientific assembly and annual meeting program. Oak Brook, Ill: Radiological Society of North America, 390
41. Gnannt R, Fischer M, Goetti R, Karlo C, Leschka S, Alkadhi H (2012) Dual-energy CT for characterization of the incidental adrenal mass: preliminary observations. AJR Am J Roentgenol 198:138–144
42. Ho LM, Marin D, Neville AM et al (2012) Characterization of adrenal nodules with dual-energy CT: Can virtual unenhanced attenuation values replace true unenhanced attenuation values? AJR Am J Roentgenol 198:840–845

43. Kim YK, Park BK, Kim CK, Park SY (2013) Adenoma characterization: adrenal protocol with dual-energy CT. Radiology 267:155–163
44. Mayo-Smith WW, Boland GW, Noto RB et al (2001) State-of-the-art adrenal imaging. Radiographics 21:995–1012
45. Slattery JM, Blake MA, Kalra MK et al (2006) Adrenocortical carcinoma: contrast wash- out characteristics on CT. AJR Am J Roentgenol 187:W21–W24

Pancreas

7

Achille Mileto, Daniele Marin and Rendon C. Nelson

7.1 Introduction

Imaging of the pancreas is challenging because of its anatomic location in the retroperitoneum and its intricate relationship with major blood vessels and bowel [1].

In the United States, acute pancreatitis, chronic pancreatitis, and pancreatic cancer are the most common pancreatic disorders [2]. Gallstone disease, which is strongly associated with obesity and the excessive consumption of alcohol, is the major risk factor for benign pancreatic disease, whereas smoking is the most important risk factor for pancreatic cancer [2].

Pancreatic cancer is a major health problem, being estimated as the fourth leading cause of cancer death in the United States and the second most common cause of death from any type of gastrointestinal disease in the world [1–3]. Pancreatic adenocarcinoma is associated with a dismal prognosis, with approximately 37,000 reported deaths in the United States in 2012 [3, 4]. In most cases, at the time of pancreatic adenocarcinoma diagnosis, metastasis or local invasion has already occurred, resulting in a low median survival of 6–12 months [3–5].

Early detection and surgical resection are the only chance of long-term survival for pancreatic cancer patients [1, 2, 4–7]. Precursor lesions of pancreatic cancer include pancreatic intra-epithelial neoplasia, intra-ductal papillary mucinous neoplasm, and mucinous cystadenoma. In addition, certain genetic predispositions are also associated with pancreatic ductal adenocarcinoma, such as a strong family history, Peutz–Jeghers syndrome, familial breast cancer syndrome, Lynch syndrome, familial atypical mole-malignant melanoma, and the *BRCA2* gene mutation [1, 2, 4–7].

Improvements in CT technology during the past decade, including fast image acquisition, improved spatial resolution, and three-dimensional renderings, have increased the accuracy of CT for pancreatic lesion detection, characterization, and staging. With single-detector CT scanners, axial imaging alone is not sufficient to demonstrate the complex anatomy of the pancreas which is optimally depicted using both multi-phasic and multi-planar imaging. MR imaging of the pancreas had an advantage over CT, because of its inherent tissue contrast, even on unenhanced images, its multi-planar capability as well as rapid serial dynamic image acquisition following the administration of intravenous contrast medium [1, 4–7]. The introduction of multi-detector CT (MDCT) in the 1990s, however, has decreased the advantages of MRI over CT. The main advantages of MDCT are the enhanced scan speed and high spatial resolution, particularly for off-axis image reconstruction, due to very thin collimation width [1, 8].

Despite continuous improvements in CT technology, the advent of reliable high-quality body magnetic resonance (MR) images, endoscopic techniques such as endoscopic ultrasound, and endoscopic retrograde cholangiopancreatography, there has been little, if any, impact on the overall

G. Ascenti et al., *CT of the Retroperitoneum*,
DOI: 10.1007/978-88-470-5469-1_7, © Springer-Verlag Italia 2014

survival of patients with pancreatic cancer [5, 6, 8–15]. Klapman [6] reported a four-decade (1965–2007) study of more than 21,000 pancreatic cancer patients from the cancer registry of Norway. In this study, the incidence and mortality from the disease remained unchanged at six to eight per 100,000. Diagnoses based on clinical findings alone decreased from 12.5 % (in the 1950s) to less than 1 % (in the 2000s), while the use of imaging techniques, such as CT and MR imaging, increased from 3.6 % to more than 30 % [5, 6].

The most widely accepted method currently advocated for screening patients at risk for development of pancreatic cancer is based on an epidemiologic approach of identifying patients at high risk for the disease [5–12]. Evaluation of this subset of patients with endoscopic ultrasound has led to the detection of pancreatic cancer in a significant number of patients at a time when surgical therapy can positively impact survival [5, 7]. However, it has proven difficult to screen for these lesions and, in general, to identify an individual at risk for the disease. For example, in most cases of pancreatic ductal adenocarcinoma , precursor lesions are not identified at screening and the disease is still diagnosed at the advanced stage [5–7, 10, 12–15].

7.2 State of the Art of Conventional (Multidetector) CT

MDCT is well established as the most accurate imaging modality for the diagnosis and staging of pancreatic lesions [10–12, 15–17]. MDCT is also the primary imaging modality for patients suspected of having a pancreatic malignancy [10–12, 15–19]. Early tumor diagnosis and accurate staging are the two most important goals for radiologists when patients suspected of having pancreatic lesion are imaged with MDCT. To accomplish these goals, MDCT must accurately reveal both local and peripancreatic invasion by tumor and the presence of liver metastases [10–19].

Since pancreatic lesions are generally isoattenuating to normal pancreatic parenchyma, unenhanced acquisition provides limited diagnostic information, unless extensive necrosis or cystic change is present (Fig. 7.1); therefore, unenhanced acquisition is currently omitted in many centers [1, 8, 12–17]. Ductal dilatation, loss of lobular texture, calcification, convexity, and irregularities of contours may be indirect signs that allow the radiologist to suspect a pancreatic tumor on unenhanced CT (Fig. 7.2). The "double duct sign," in which a tumor obstructs both the pancreatic and contiguous extrahepatic common bile ducts, is a reliable indicator of an obstructing lesion (Fig. 7.3), although it is not entirely specific for pancreatic adenocarcinoma [1, 8, 12–17, 20]. Tumors in the head and body of the pancreas frequently cause main pancreatic duct obstruction with upstream ductal dilatation and, over time, parenchymal atrophy (Fig. 7.4) [1, 17–20]. Conversely, small tumors in the uncinate process are very often inconspicuous on CT and loss of the pancreatic contour may be the only abnormality. Tumors of the uncinate process are associated with a poor prognosis, when there is a delayed clinical presentation due to close proximity and early involvement of the superior mesenteric vessels [1, 17–21]. Although unenhanced images can provide baseline attenuation measurements for focal lesions and allow comparison with contrast-enhanced images for lesion enhancement, this information is of limited diagnostic utility [1, 8, 12–20].

The administration of intravenous contrast material is a crucial requirement in MDCT protocols for pancreatic lesion evaluation. Contrast-enhanced CT has a sensitivity ranging from 89 to 97 % for tumor detection and a positive predictive value of 89–100 % for determining tumor unresectability [1, 8]. To maximize the conspicuity of vessels and pancreatic tumors, the pancreas and adjacent visceral structures are commonly scanned during different phases of contrast enhancement. In general, a biphasic CT study of the pancreas, consisting of pancreatic parenchymal and venous phase acquisitions, is currently the accepted technique for the detection

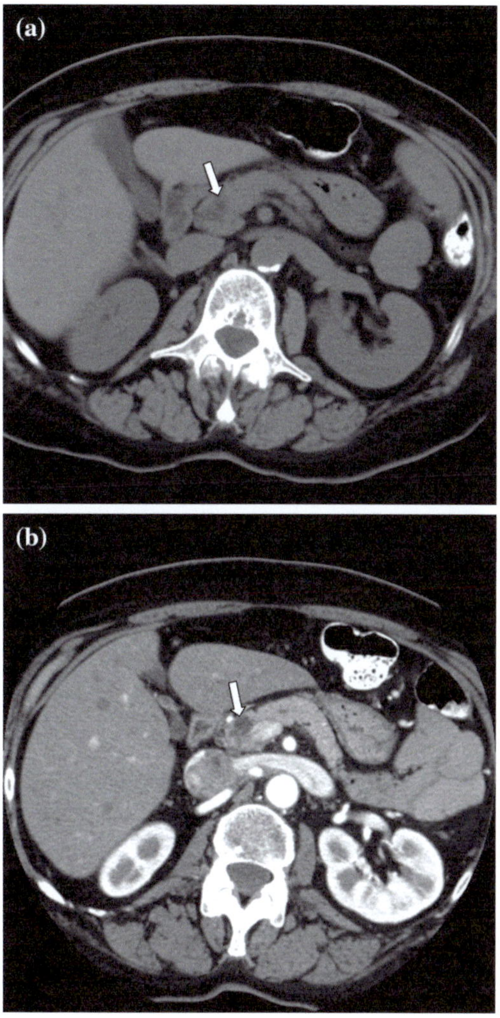

Fig. 7.1 Intra-ductal papillary mucinous neoplasm of the pancreatic head. The lesion (*arrow*) appears slightly hypodense to normal pancreatic parenchyma on the unenhanced image (**a**) and is well identifiable on the contrast-enhanced pancreatic parenchymal phase image (**b**)

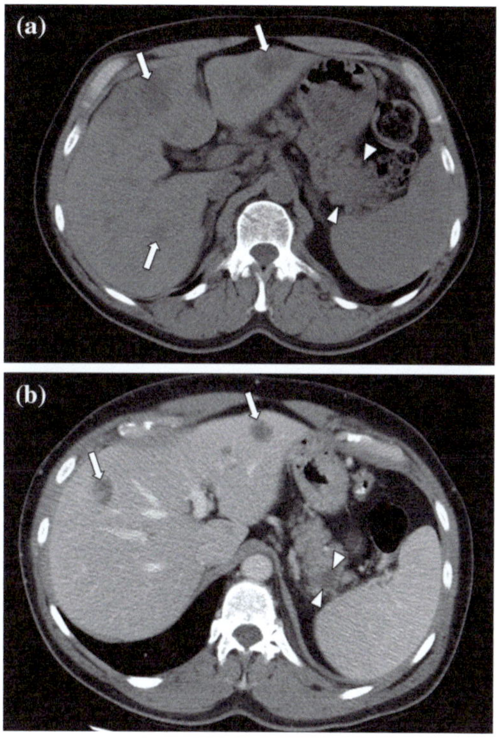

Fig. 7.2 Adenocarcinoma of the pancreatic tail. An enlargement of the pancreatic tail, associated with loss of lobular texture, convexity, and irregularities of contours (*arrowheads*), is visible on the unenhanced image (**a**); multiple hepatic hypodense lesions (*arrows*) are also visible. Contrast-enhanced portal venous phase image (**b**) clearly shows a hypodense solid lesion (*arrowheads*) in the pancreatic tail with associated hepatic metastases (*arrows*)

and staging of pancreatic ductal adenocarcinoma (Fig. 7.5) [21–29]. Note that the pancreatic parenchymal phase occurs approximately 10–15 s later than the late hepatic arterial phase used for hypervascular liver lesion detection. In particular, with the use of modern bolus-tracking timing techniques, it starts with a delay of about 17–18 s after arrival of the bolus in the abdominal aorta at predefined attenuation threshold of 100 HU.

With CT, pancreatic adenocarcinoma typically appears hypoenhancing relative to the pancreatic parenchyma on early phase images and becomes less conspicuity compared to the adjacent pancreatic parenchyma on venous phase images (Fig. 7.6). This enhancement pattern is likely related to the desmoplasia and fibrosis, typically present within malignant pancreatic tumors [1, 8, 12, 15–17, 21–28]. Conversely, islet cell tumors, accounting for about 5 % of all pancreatic neoplasms, are generally small hyperenhancing masses that lack associated desmoplastic reaction [15–17, 21–28].

In terms of the diagnostic performance of multi-phasic CT for the detection of pancreatic tumors, initially there was no agreement on

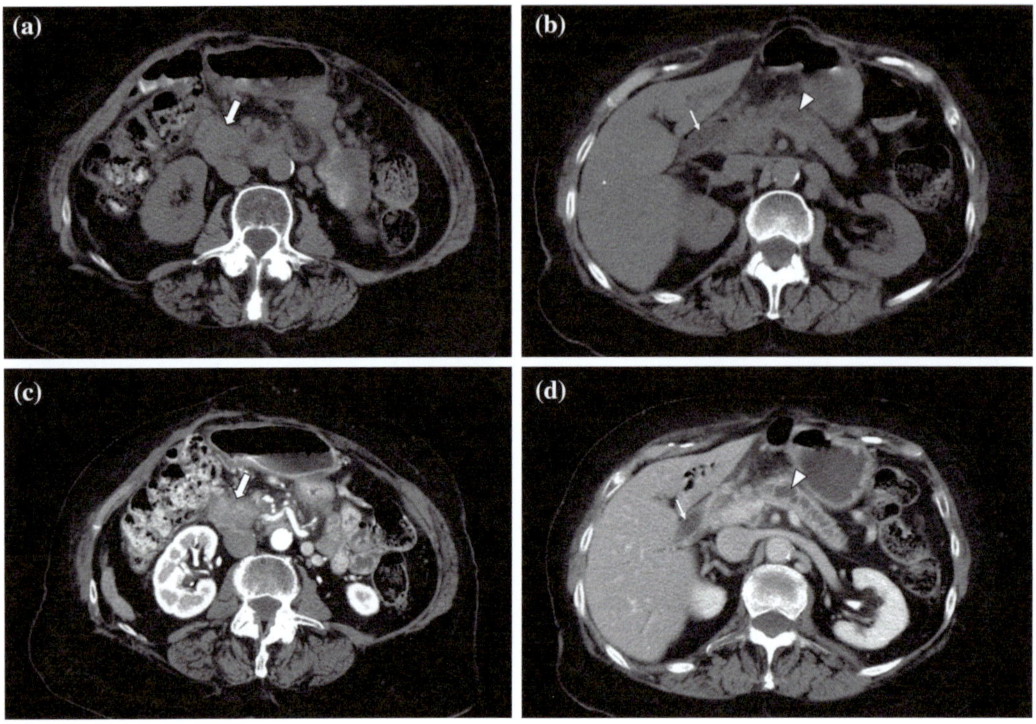

Fig. 7.3 Adenocarcinoma of the pancreatic head. Unenhanced (**a, b**), contrast-enhanced pancreatic parenchymal- (**c**), and portal venous (**d**) phase images show an enlargement of the inferior portion of the pancreatic head, with convexity and irregularities of contours (*arrow*), with dilatation of both the pancreatic (*arrowhead*) and common bile ducts (*thin arrow*) ("double duct sign")

timing of the arterial phase acquisition [1, 8, 12, 15–17, 21–28]. Choi et al. [22, 30] reported that tumor detectability on arterial phase images obtained starting at 30 s after the initiation of contrast material was superior (95 %) to that on portal venous phase images obtained at 80 s (68 %). Conversely, Keogan [16] and Graf [17] reported that arterial phase images, when added to portal venous phase images, did not contribute to the improvement in the detection of pancreatic adenocarcinomas [16, 17, 22]. Meanwhile, Lu et al. first [18] introduced a new concept: pancreatic parenchymal phase imaging. This study suggested that the arterial phase images should be obtained beginning at 40 s after the initiation of contrast material during the so-called pancreatic parenchymal phase. This phase of enhancement consistently yields the highest lesion detection rate with optimal tumor conspicuity. The rationale for this observation is that CT images are acquired during peak pancreatic enhancement, when the maximum difference in attenuation is attained between poorly vascularized pancreatic tumors and vividly enhancing pancreatic parenchyma (Fig. 7.7) [18, 22]. Moreover, adequate mesenteric venous and arterial opacification for detection of vascular invasion is achieved during the pancreatic parenchymal phase of enhancement [29].

Nowadays, most authors state that the initial phase of a contrast-enhanced biphasic pancreatic examination should be the pancreatic parenchymal phase (Fig. 7.8) [18, 29, 31]. Only a few authors advocate that the initial phase of the biphasic examination should be an earlier arterial phase [15–17]. The earlier arterial phase is reliable for depicting hyperenhancing lesions (i.e., most islet cell neuroendocrine tumors), which typically have early peak enhancement and rapid washout. However, since most islet cell tumors

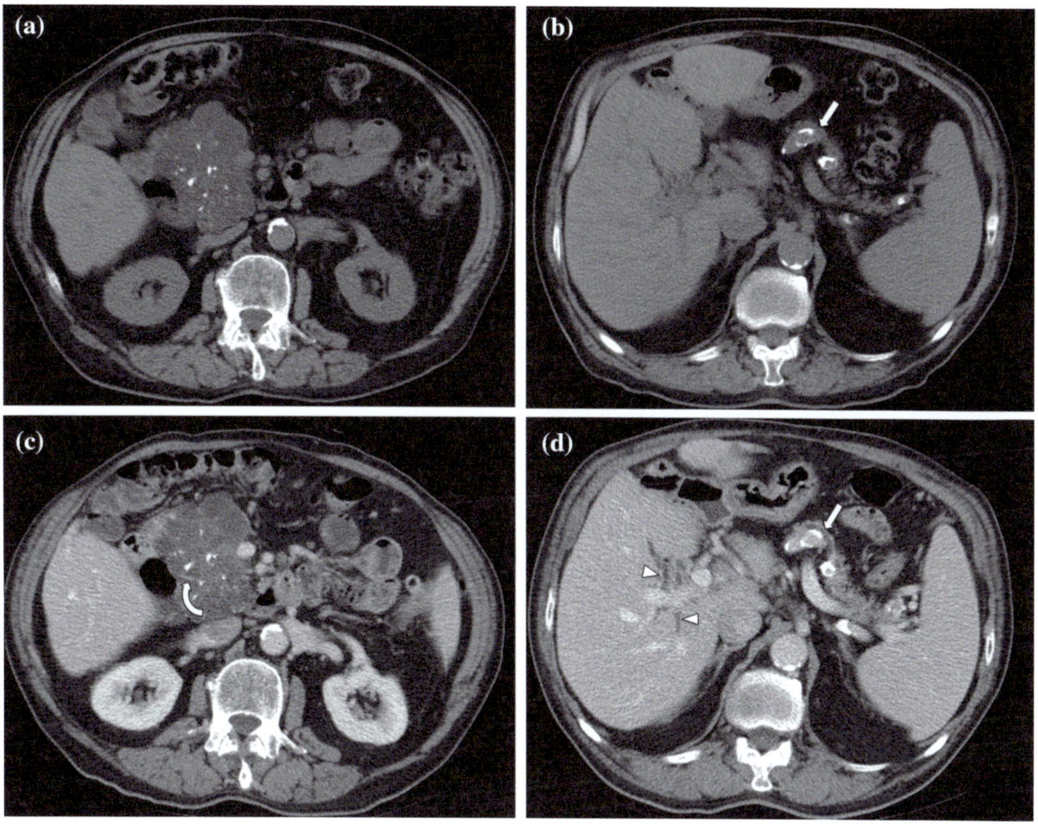

Fig. 7.4 Serous cystadenoma of the pancreatic head. Unenhanced images (**a, b**) show a large multi-locular mass with multiple internal calcification within the pancreatic head (**a**), associated with upstream pancreatic main duct dilatation (*arrow*) and parenchymal atrophy (**b**). Contrast-enhanced portal venous phase images (**c, d**) better depict some enhancing septations (*curved arrow*) within the mass (**c**), upstream pancreatic main duct dilatation (*arrow*) as well as intra-hepatic biliary duct dilation (*arrowheads*) (**d**)

are also confidently identified during the pancreatic parenchymal phase, it is not necessary to have two different CT protocols [28, 29]. For this reason, there is general agreement that when a biphasic dynamic CT is performed, the earlier phase should be performed during the pancreatic parenchymal phase [14, 15].

Some centers use a small field of view to improve in-plane (x-axis and y-axis) spatial resolution and aid detection of small masses during the pancreatic parenchymal phase [8, 32]. This strategy has two important drawbacks: (1) exclusion of the outer portions of the liver, which must be evaluated for early-enhancing metastases particularly from an islet cell tumor, and (2) increased image noise due to the use of small voxels which may obscure small or subtle lesions [8].

The portal venous phase, during which there is maximum hepatic parenchymal enhancement, is usually performed as the later phase of a contrast-enhanced biphasic pancreas protocol. Imaging during the portal venous phase (70–90 s after the initiation of contrast material) provides optimal detection of hypoenhancing hepatic metastases from pancreatic adenocarcinoma as well as distant metastases and other ancillary findings such as lymph nodes, peritoneal implants, and malignant ascites (Figs. 7.9, 7.10, 7.11) [1, 4–8, 10–21]. The other advantage of imaging during the portal venous phase is the optimal delineation of the portal, splenic, and superior mesenteric veins

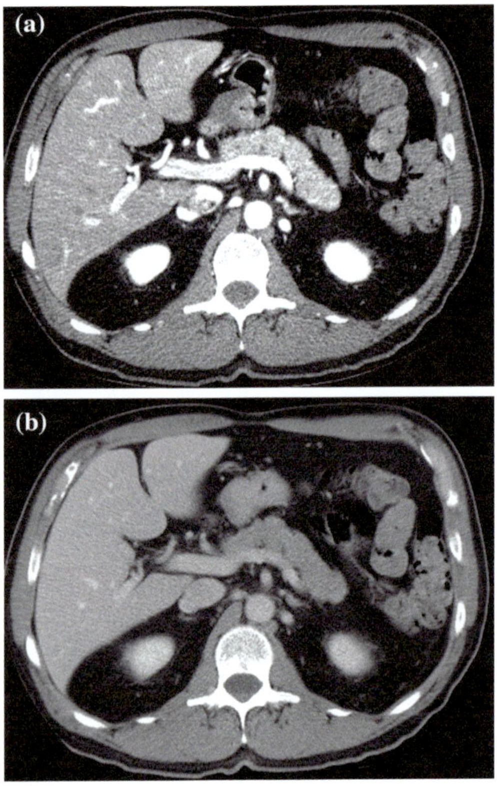

Fig. 7.5 Example of contrast-enhanced biphasic MDCT study of the pancreas, consisting of contrast-enhanced pancreatic parenchymal (**a**) and portal venous (**c**) phase images. Note that the pancreatic parenchyma is homogeneously and vividly enhancing during the pancreatic parenchymal phase (**a**), whereas a homogeneous decrease in the parenchymal enhancement degree is appreciable during the portal venous phase (**b**)

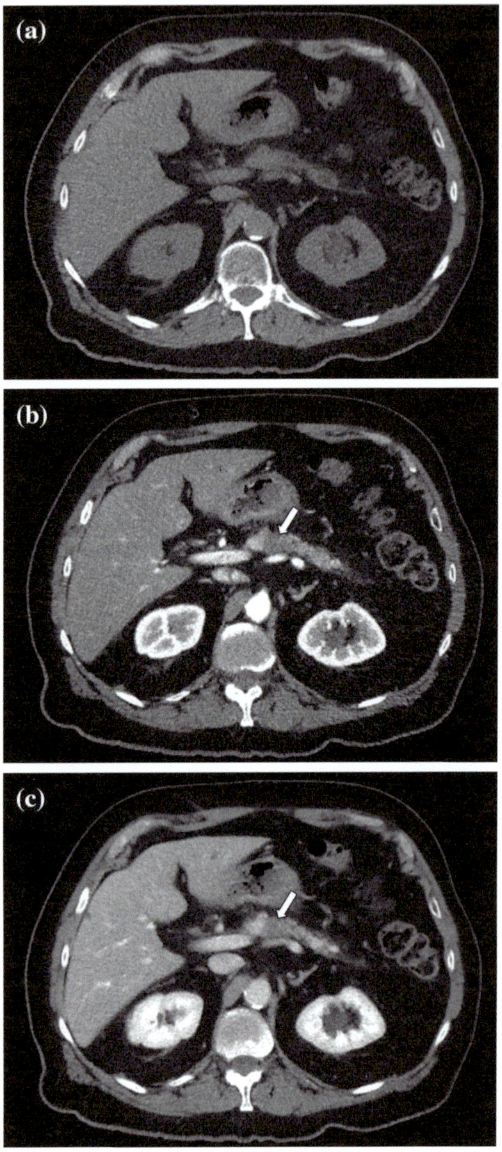

Fig. 7.6 Adenocarcinoma of the pancreatic body. The lesion is isodense to normal pancreatic parenchyma and therefore poorly identifiable on unenhanced image (**a**). By exploiting the maximum difference in attenuation between the poorly vascularized lesion and vividly enhancing pancreatic parenchyma, contrast-enhanced pancreatic parenchymal phase image (**b**) clearly shows a small lesion (*arrow*) in the pancreatic body. Although the tumor continues to be visible on the portal venous phase image (*arrow*) (**c**), the tumor conspicuity is lower compared to the pancreatic parenchymal phase image (**b**)

[1, 8, 12–20, 25–28]. Thrombosis of the portal vein is a common complication of pancreatic adenocarcinoma, and determination of patency versus invasion has important implications for the resectability of pancreatic masses [8, 20]. Moreover, this study phase provides a second look at the pancreas, which may be helpful on occasion [1, 4–8, 10–21].

After a pancreatic lesion is detected, the second goal for the radiologist interpreting the CT is preoperative tumor staging and likelihood of tumor resectability at surgery. In the absence of hepatic metastases or local tumor extension (i.e., invasion

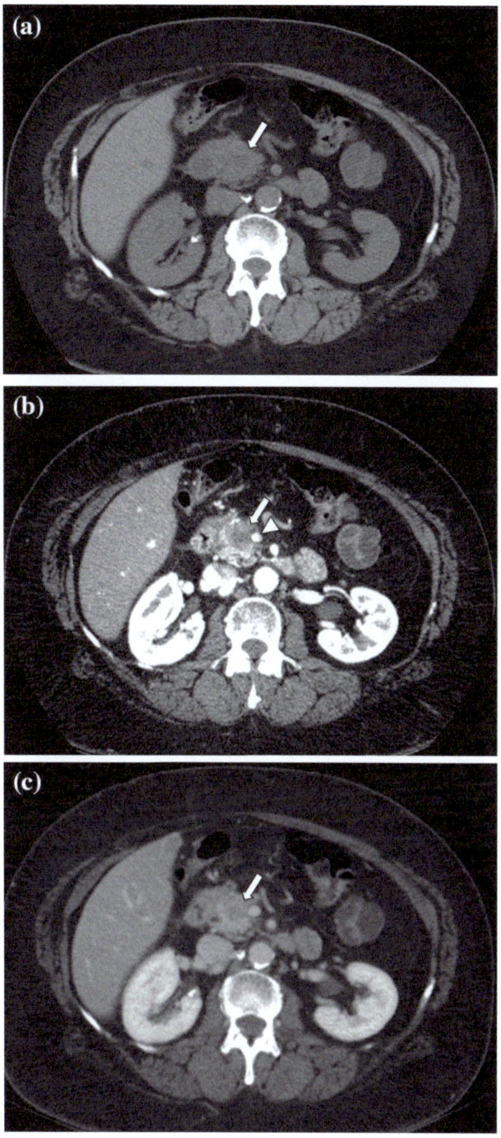

Fig. 7.7 Adenocarcinoma of the pancreatic head. An enlargement of the pancreatic head, associated with loss of lobular texture, convexity, and irregularities of contours (*arrow*), is visible on the unenhanced image (**a**). The pancreatic parenchymal phase image (**b**) clearly shows a hypodense mass (*arrow*) within the pancreatic head; the mass encases nearly 180° of the superior mesenteric artery (*arrowhead*). The mass (*arrow*) is ill-defined on the portal venous phase image (**c**)

of adjacent organs), tumor resectability will depend on the presence of vascular involvement [33]. The superior mesenteric artery (SMA) is the most common artery involved in carcinoma of the pancreas, particularly for lesions arising from the pancreatic head (Fig. 7.12) [33, 34]. The celiac artery and its major branches are also frequently involved in pancreatic cancer, especially in larger tumors and in tumors of the pancreatic body and tail [33–35]. Arterial involvement significantly reduces the success of curative surgical resection [33]. Notably, limited tumor involvement of smaller arterial branches, such as the pancreaticoduodenal and gastroduodenal arteries, is generally not considered an absolute contraindication to surgery (Fig. 7.9) [33–35]. MDCT has an overall negative predictive value of 100 % for predicting vascular invasion, and a CT grading system of vascular involvement has been reported by Lu et al. [1, 36]. These authors prospectively graded vessel involvement using a 0- to 4-point scale based on the degree of circumferential contiguity of the tumor to the vessel (Grade 0: no contiguity, Grade 1: <25 % contiguity, Grade 2: 25–50 % contiguity, Grade 3: 50–75 % contiguity, Grade 4: >75 % contiguity) (Fig. 7.13). They found that when more than 50 % of the vessel's circumference (grades 3 and 4) was in contact with a vessel, the likelihood of successful tumor resection was low [36], with a sensitivity and specificity for unresectability of 84 and 98 %, respectively [33–36].

The assessment of venous structures such as the portal vein, superior mesenteric vein, and splenic vein also plays an important role in determining the feasibility of surgery in patients with pancreatic cancer. The CT grading system described by Lu et al. [36] can be also applied to veins [33, 36, 37]. Unequivocal invasion of the venous wall by tumor, rather than simple contiguity, is generally necessary to assess resectability. Tumor involvement of larger veins, such as the portal vein and/or superior mesenteric vein, is generally regarded as a contraindication for surgery. Isolated involvement of the proximal (upstream) portal vein, however, will not necessarily preclude pancreatic surgery as some institutions will follow tumor resection with a venous graft reconstruction [37].

Lymphatic channels within the pancreas drain into lymph nodes around the celiac axis and the superior mesenteric vein. As these lymphatic vessels become engorged with tumor cells, they

Study phase	Timing	Findings
Unenhanced phase	Before contrast medium administration	Ductal dilatation, loss of lobular texture, calcification, convexity, irregularities of glandular contours, tumor baseline measurements
Pancreatic parenchymal phase	40 s after contrast medium administration	Hypo- and hyperenhancing lesion detection, tumor staging, (vascular anatomy and locoregional assessment)
Portal venous phase	70-90 s after contrast medium administration	Tumor staging (venous patency and hepatic mestases)

Fig. 7.8 Summary of pancreatic MDCT acquisition protocol [8]

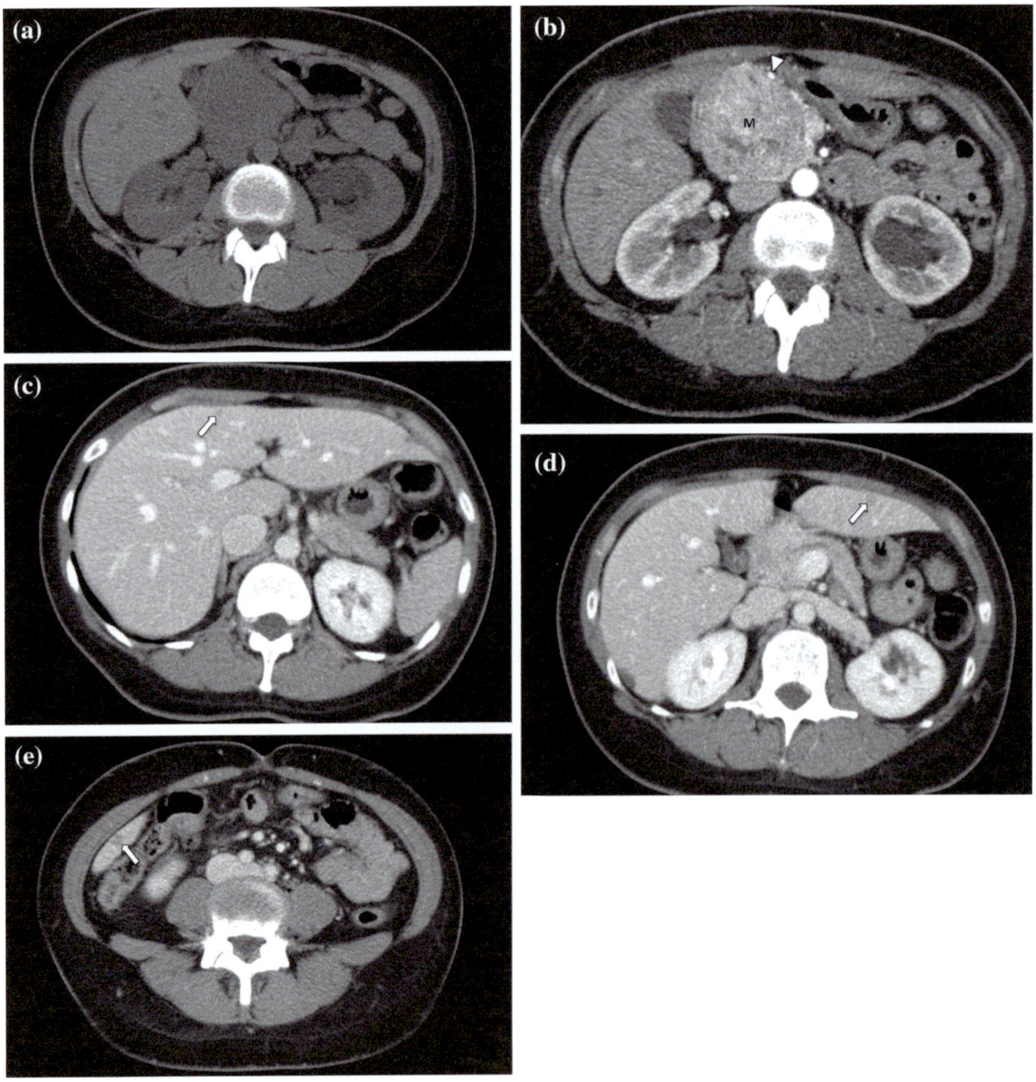

Fig. 7.9 Neuroendocrine tumor of the pancreatic head. An enlargement of the pancreatic head, associated with loss of lobular texture, convexity, and irregularities of contours (*arrow*), is visible on the unenhanced image (**a**). The mass (*M*) is vividly and heterogeneously enhancing on the pancreatic parenchymal phase image (**b**); note encasement of the gastroduodenal artery (*arrowhead*). Portal venous phase images (**c–e**) show multiple small hepatic metastases (*arrows*)

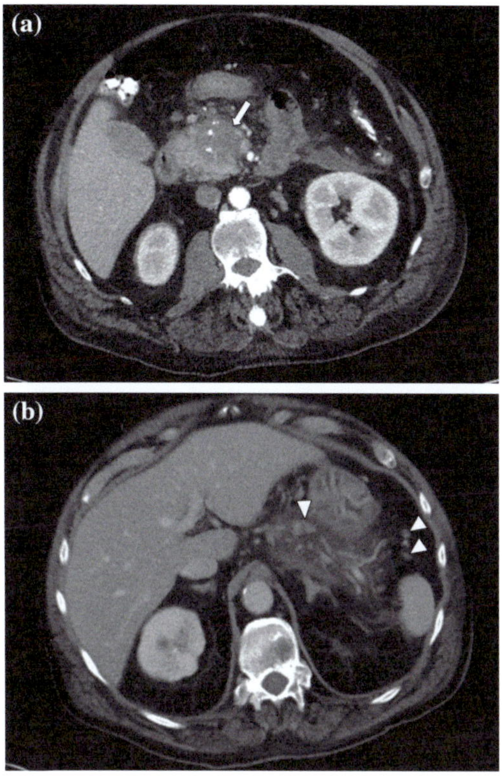

Fig. 7.10 Adenocarcinoma of the pancreatic head. Pancreatic parenchymal phase image (**a**) shows a hypoenhancing mass (*arrow*) with internal calcifications in the pancreatic head. Portal venous phase image (**b**) shows peripancreatic lymph nodes (*arrowheads*)

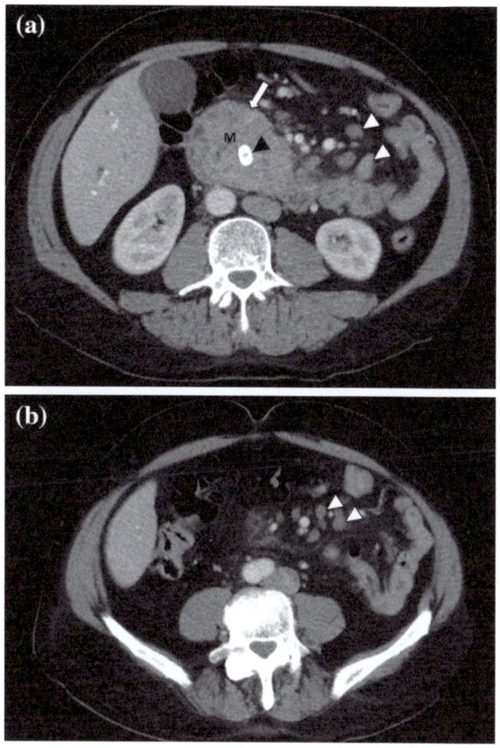

Fig. 7.11 a, b Adenocarcinoma of the pancreatic head. Portal venous phase image through the pancreatic head shows a large and moderately enhancing mass. Note the presence of a metallic biliary stent (*black arrowhead*) and several peripancreatic lymph nodes (*white arrowheads*)

produce a perivascular cuff of soft tissue that represents extrapancreatic disease [20]. On occasion, this perivascular cuff may be the only radiologic sign of a pancreatic carcinoma [20]. The assessment of lymph nodes in pancreatic tumors deserves a special mention. CT is inaccurate for the detection of regional lymph node metastases [1, 40–42]. The CT criteria for nodal involvement, based on size, are less reliable as large lymph nodes may be hyperplastic and normal-sized lymph nodes may have microscopic metastases. The low detection rate of regional lymph node metastases has limited clinical implications, as peripancreatic lymph nodes are routinely resected at surgery [1, 40–42]. Moreover, regional lymph node metastasis is not a contraindication for surgical resection if there is no evidence of vascular invasion or distant metastases [1, 40–43].

Three-dimensional volume display of CT angiographic datasets also provides a comprehensive display of the key arterial and venous anatomy needed to properly determine resectability of pancreatic cancer [33]. Curved planar reformatting (CPR) , maximum intensity projection (MIP), or volume rendering can be particularly advantageous for evaluating the peripancreatic vasculature (Fig. 7.14) [33–35, 38].

Finally, the staging of pancreatic lesions should always provide information about hepatic metastases, local tumor extension to the adjacent viscera, such as stomach and colon, and peritoneal deposits. All these features preclude surgical resection [38, 39].

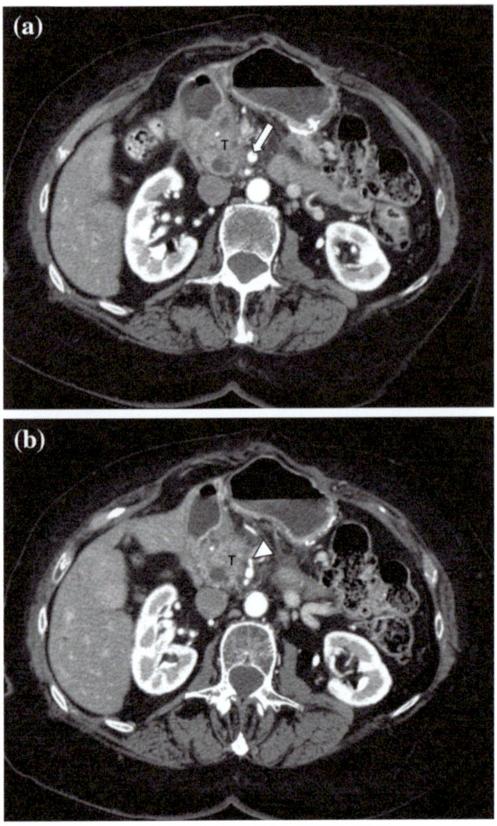

Fig. 7.12 Adenocarcinoma of the pancreatic head. Pancreatic parenchymal phase images (**a, b**) show a hypoenhancing mass in the head of the pancreas (*T*) with Grade 2 (<180°) tumor encasement of the right side of the superior mesenteric artery, as well as on the proximal branches (*arrowhead*)

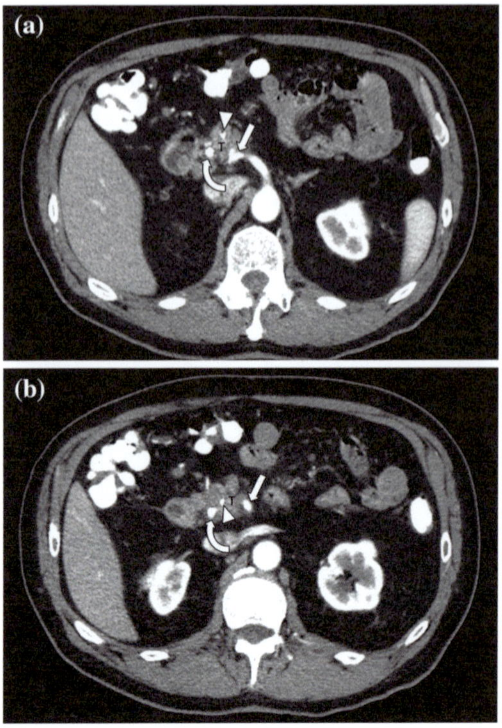

Fig. 7.13 Adenocarcinoma of the pancreatic head. Pancreatic parenchymal phase images (**a, b**) show Grade 2 (90–180°) contiguity of the tumor (*T*) with the proximal superior mesenteric artery (*arrow*). Note the presence of common bile duct (*curved arrow*) and main pancreatic duct stents (*arrowhead*)

Despite the developments of new-generation MDCT scanners, approximately 11 % of pancreatic ductal adenocarcinomas still remain undetected by CT because of the lack of a visible attenuation difference between the lesion and the adjacent pancreatic parenchyma. These lesions may be detectable only by identification of a contour abnormality or segmental dilation of the pancreatic duct [9].

Some CT imaging issues such as radiation dose and image quality have also to be considered in pancreatic imaging. In particular, radiologists must carefully weigh dose concerns ("delivering as low radiation dose as possible") against issues of image quality [8]. As in other body CT applications, one strategy for decreasing the radiation dose is to reduce the number of study phases. Imbriaco et al. [44] described a single-phase CT protocol for pancreatic lesion detection using a scan delay of 50 s from the beginning of contrast medium administration. These authors found this approach to be effective for the diagnosis and assessment of resectability of patients with suspected pancreatic adenocarcinoma , with the advantages of being less time-consuming, having fewer images to store, and reducing the radiation dose to patients [44, 45]. Another approach to reducing the radiation dose is by modulating the tube current according to the patient's size. Automatic tube current modulation, which adjusts CT tube current according to preset measures of desired image quality, is available on all modern CT systems [46–48]. Recently, Marin et al. [46] demonstrated that

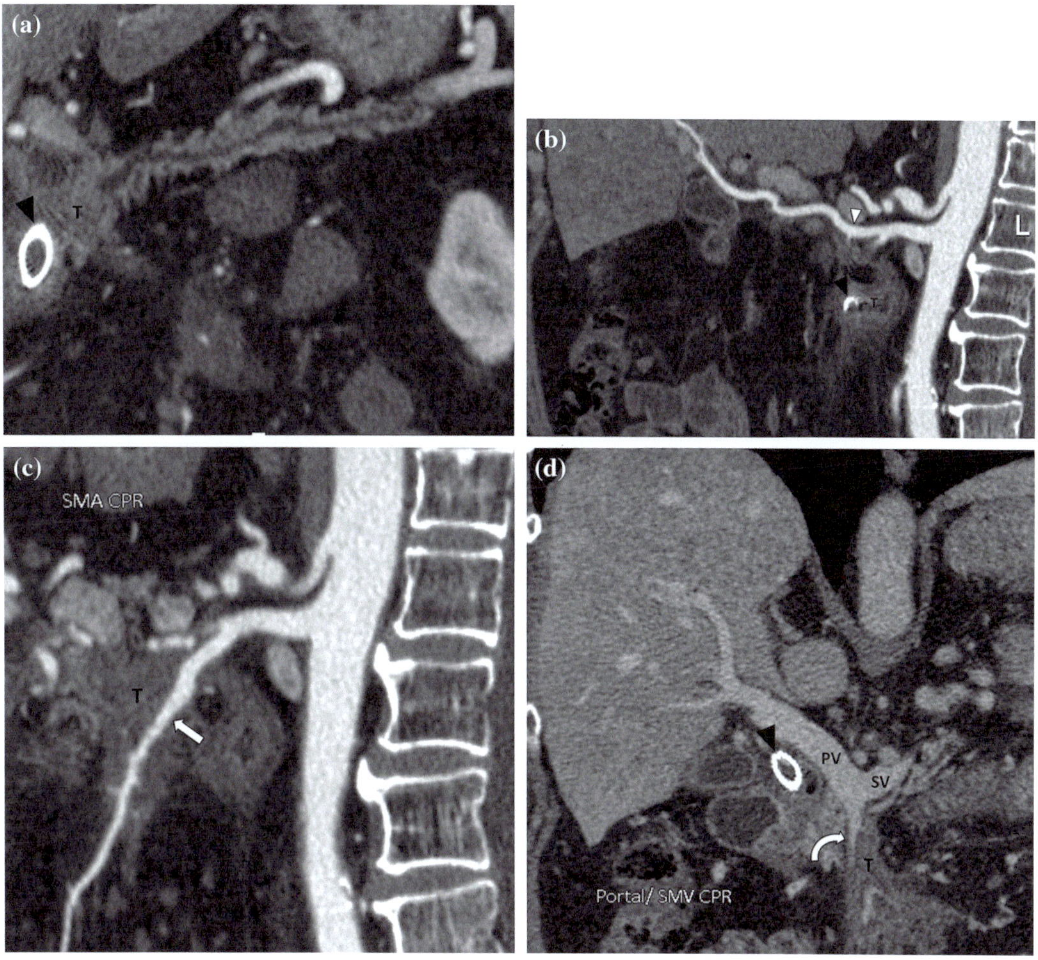

Fig. 7.14 Benefits of a CPR image in advanced adenocarcinoma of the pancreatic head. Pancreatic parenchymal phase CPR image through the pancreas (**a**) shows the presence of a tumor (*T*) in the pancreatic head with upstream main pancreatic duct dilatation. Note the presence of a metallic stent in the common bile duct (*black arrowhead*). Pancreatic parenchymal phase CPR image through the course of the right hepatic artery (**b**) depicts perivascular tumor extension (*arrowhead*). Note that in this patient, the right hepatic artery arises from the superior mesenteric artery, whereas the left hepatic artery arises from the celiac trunk. Pancreatic parenchymal phase CPR image (**c**) through the course of the superior mesenteric artery (*arrow*) shows Grade 4 (>270°) contiguity of the tumor (*T*). Portal venous phase CPR image (**d**) through the portal confluence also depicts >270° contiguity of the tumor with the superior mesenteric vein (*curved arrow*). The portal vein (*PV*) and the splenic vein (*SV*) are not involved

compared with a high-tube-voltage CT protocol (140 kVp), a low-tube-voltage (80 kVp), high-tube-current (675 mA) CT technique has the potential for improving the enhancement of the pancreas and peripancreatic vasculature, improving tumor conspicuity, and reducing patient radiation dose during the pancreatic parenchymal phase. In addition, new iterative reconstruction techniques can provide improved image quality from noisier source datasets, allowing a further reduction in the radiation dose [8, 46–50]. Some recent studies have suggested that compared with a standard filtered back-projection reconstruction algorithm, the use of iterative reconstruction algorithms can lead to significantly improved image quality and enables lower radiation dose acquisitions on MDCT scanners [49–51].

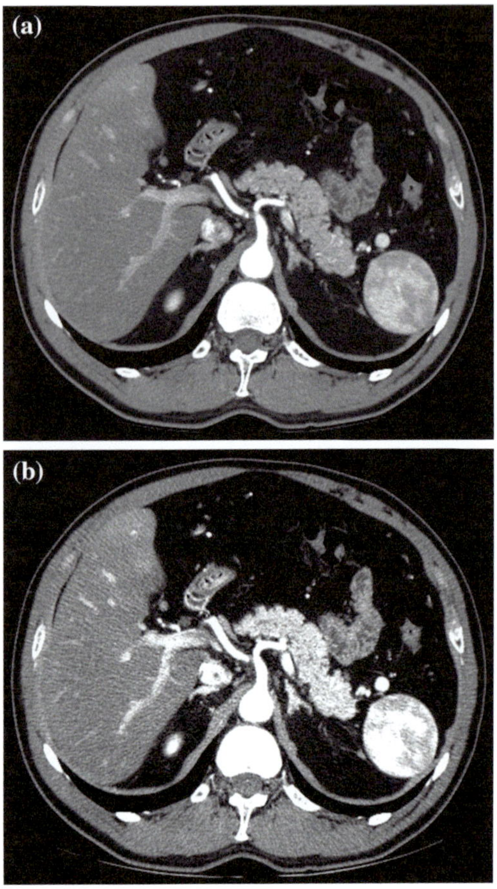

Fig. 7.15 Benefits of 80- versus 140-kVp tube voltage setting. Compared with the high-kVp image (**a**), the 80-kVp image (**b**) demonstrates superior enhancement of both the pancreas and peripancreatic vasculature

7.3 Spectral CT: Study Protocols and Clinical Applications

Spectral CT has specific clinical applications for imaging of pancreatic lesions.

Firstly, tumor-to-pancreas contrast and lesion conspicuity, key determinants of sensitivity, can benefit from low-tube-voltage, high-tube-current settings. The reason for this observation is that there is an increase in photoelectric absorption and a decrease in Compton scatter when CT is performed using lower photon energies such as 80 kVp rather than at 120 or 140 kVp. The photoelectric effect occurs primarily with elements that have a higher atomic number such as iodine. As a result, the attenuation of iodinated contrast media is significantly higher at a lower kVp [46, 47, 52–54]. Based on this assumption, CT scans obtained with 80-kVp photons generated during a dual-energy acquisition demonstrate higher conspicuity of a hypovascular and therefore hypoenhancing pancreatic neoplasm compared to the vividly enhancing adjacent pancreatic parenchyma [46, 47, 52–54]. This advantage can be clinically exploited during both the pancreatic parenchymal and portal venous phases of enhancement.

Recent studies [46, 55] have demonstrated that imaging at 80 kVp results in significantly higher contrast enhancement of the pancreas and a greater pancreas-to-tumor contrast-to-noise ratio during the pancreatic parenchymal phase of enhancement. Marin et al. [46] showed that compared with high-kVp settings, single-energy pancreatic imaging with a tube voltage setting of 80 kVp improves the enhancement of both pancreas and peripancreatic vasculatures (Fig. 7.15). In this study, the estimated effective radiation dose decreased from 18.5 to 5.1 mSv, at the cost of slightly higher image noise for 80 kVp compared with 140 kVp, with a mean dose saving of 71 % [46, 55].

Another recent study [55] demonstrated that pancreatic spectral CT improves tumor conspicuity on images interpreted at lower viewing energies, particularly when viewed at the individual patients' optimal contrast-to-noise ratio. This advantage has the potential to allow better detection of small, early, and/or isoattenuating pancreatic lesions. Viewing images at the optimal contrast-to-noise ratio may also offer the benefits of improved lesion conspicuity without degradation of image quality from the image noise associated with the lowest energies (Fig. 7.16) [55].

Other authors [52, 57] have suggested that the benefits of spectral CT can be exploited by performing dual-energy scanning during the portal venous phase of enhancement instead of the pancreatic parenchymal phase. The advantage of spectral CT during the portal venous phase is related to the inherently lower

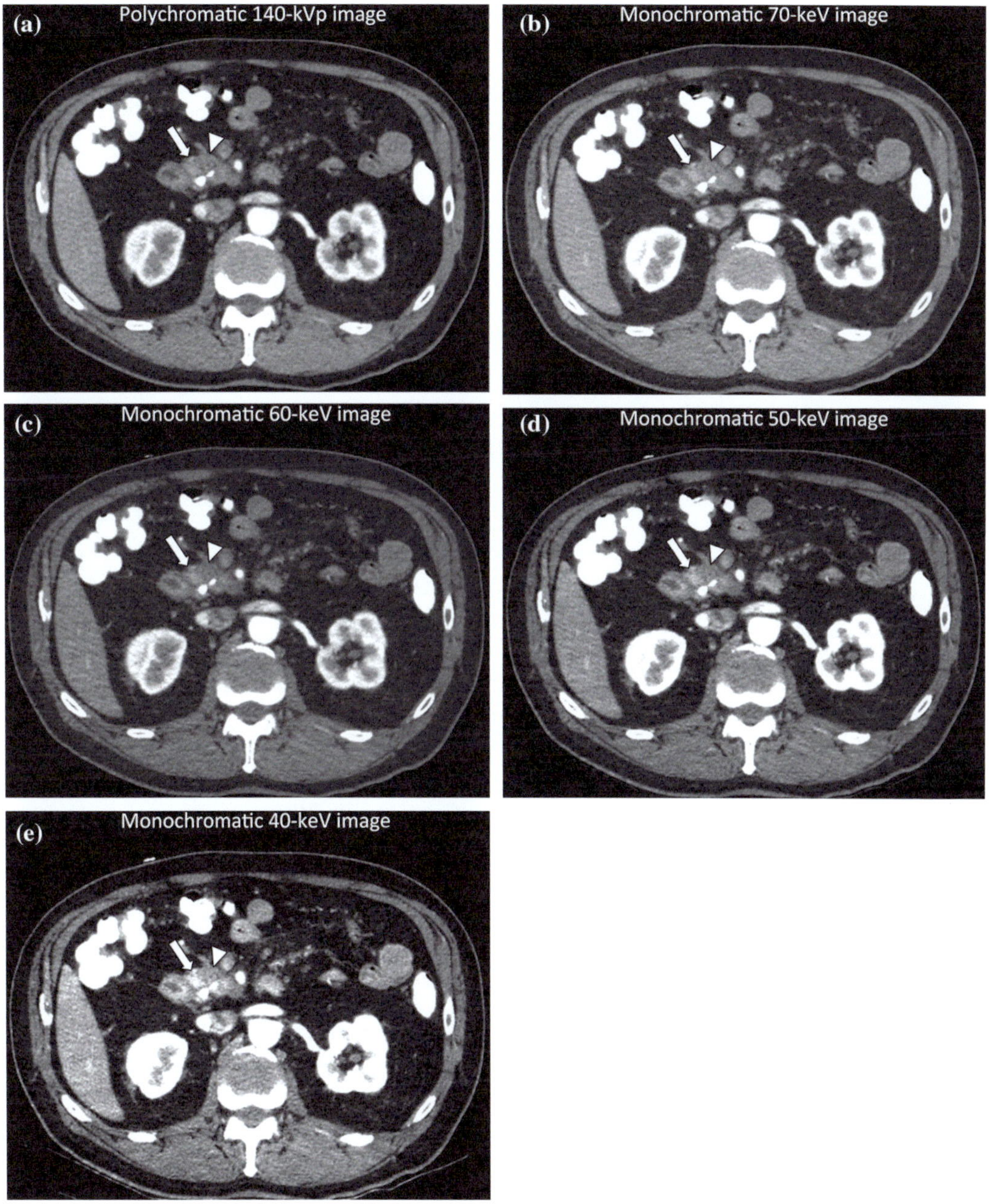

Fig. 7.16 **a–e** Comparison between polychromatic 140-kVp and monochromatic 70-, 60-, 50-, and 40-keV images in a patient with adenocarcinoma of the pancreatic head. Note that as the monochromatic energy level is lowered, there is improved differentiation between normal pancreatic parenchyma (*arrow*) and the tumor (*arrowhead*)

enhancement or attenuation differences between malignant pancreatic tumors and adjacent normal parenchyma during this phase, particularly when compared to a 120-kVp dataset [52, 57]. Moreover, contrast-to-noise ratio , subjective assessment of malignant pancreatic tumors, and

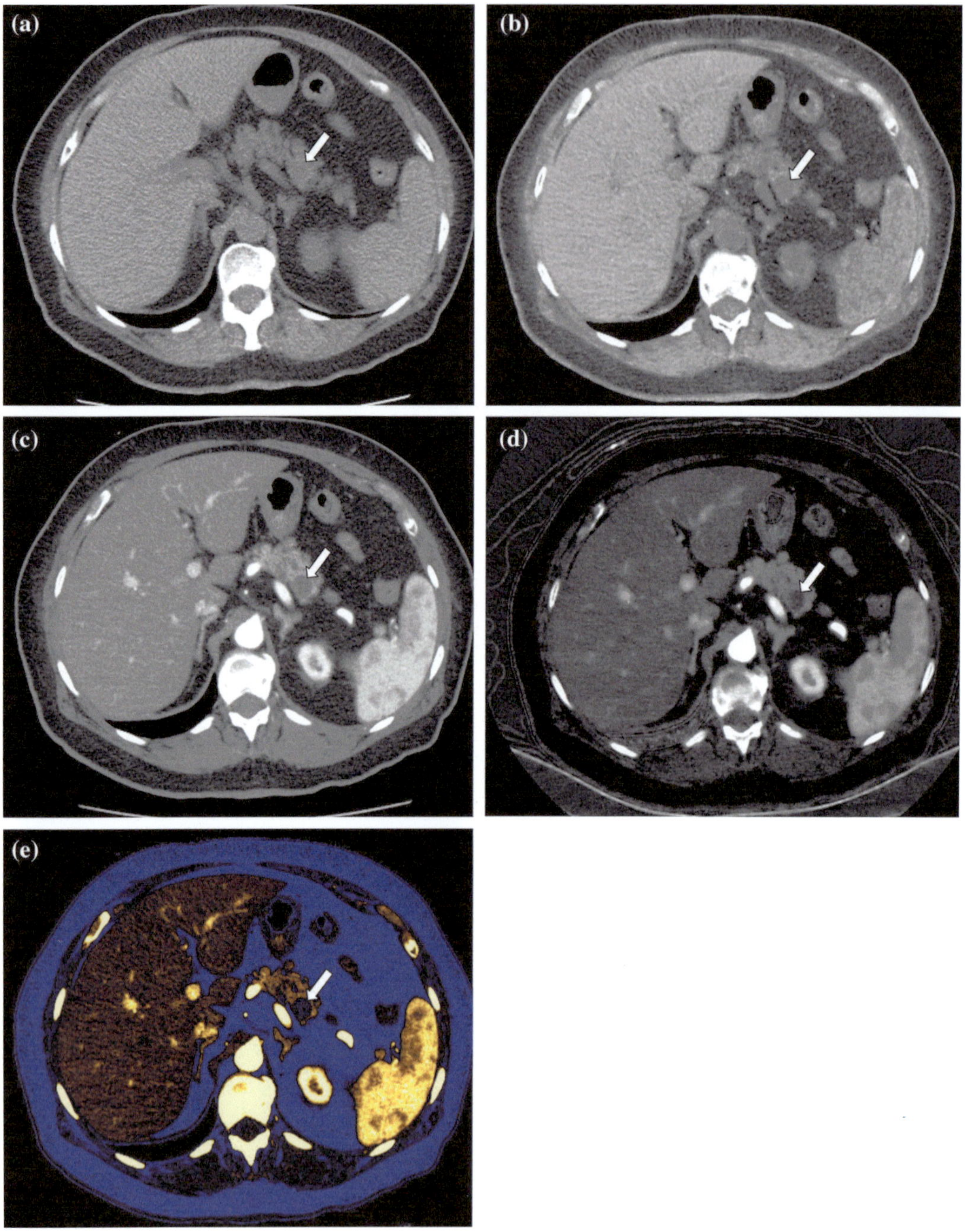

Fig. 7.17 Example of spectral CT workflow in a patient with a side branch intra-ductal papillary mucinous neoplasm (*IPMN*) of the pancreatic tail. The lesion (*arrow*) is slightly visible on both standard (**a**) and virtual unenhanced (**b**) images. Note that the virtual unenhanced (**b**) and standard unenhanced images (**a**) can be easily discriminated, since virtual unenhanced appears slightly more grainy than conventional unenhanced series due to smoothing induced by the post-processing algorithm. The lesion (*arrow*) is clearly visible on both 140-kVp (**c**) and iodine-density images (**d**). Further advantages are provided by color-coded iodine overlay image (**e**) which shows a color void of iodine signal within the lesion (*arrow*)

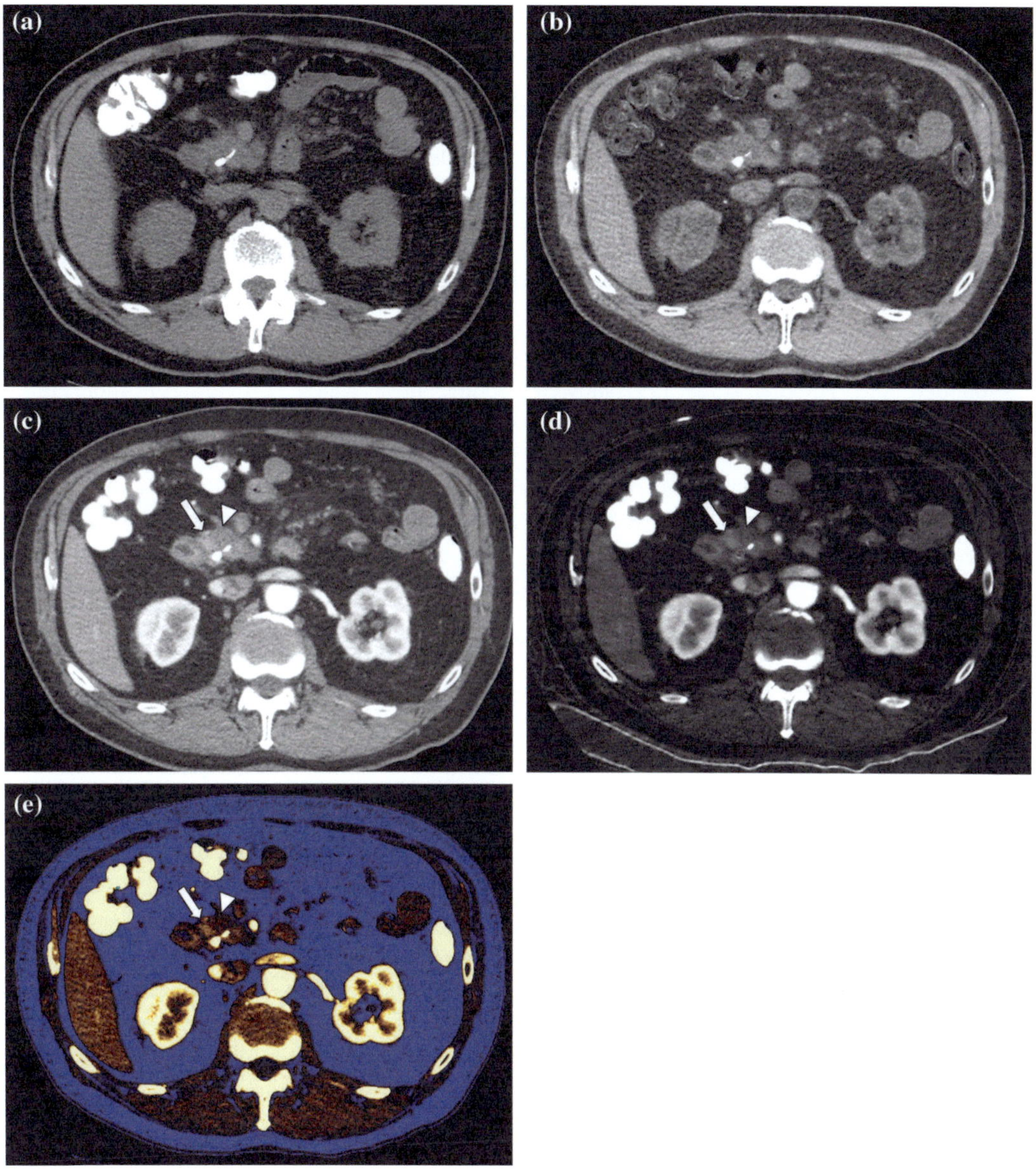

Fig. 7.18 Example of spectral CT workflow in a patient with adenocarcinoma of the pancreatic head (same case as Fig. 7.16). The lesion is isoattenuating to normal pancreatic parenchyma on both standard (**a**) and virtual unenhanced (**b**) images. Note that the virtual unenhanced image (**b**) closely approximates the standard unenhanced image (**a**). The lesion (*arrowhead*) is clearly differentiated from normal parenchyma (*arrow*) on both 140-kVp (**c**) and iodine-density images (**d**). Based on different degrees of iodine uptake, as shown in the color-coded iodine overlay image (**e**), there is improved differentiation of the hypovascular lesion (*arrowhead*) from the highly vascularized normal parenchyma (*arrow*)

pancreatic duct visualization are significantly better at 80 kVp compared to 120 kVp [52, 57]. One of these studies [52, 57] concluded that it is possible to significantly reduce the radiation dose to patients if the pancreas is scanned in dual-energy mode during the portal venous phase of enhancement. The authors hypothesized that two separate acquisitions may no longer be needed if tumor conspicuity is maintained during the portal venous phase of enhancement at 80 kVp, thus potentially eliminating the need for the pancreatic parenchymal phase [52, 57].

More recently, a study was published demonstrating the added diagnostic value of spectral-based virtual unenhanced and iodine-only images for evaluation of pancreatic tumors, especially for determining the cystic or solid nature of pancreatic tumors (Fig. 7.17) [58]. A calculated mean radiation dose saving of 14 % was achieved if the standard unenhanced dataset was omitted [58]. Another study [59] showed that virtual unenhanced images from a dual-energy dataset acquired during the pancreatic parenchymal phase demonstrated no significant difference in image quality and provided less image noise than true unenhanced imaging. This study also showed that a radiation dose saving of about 27 % can be achieved if standard unenhanced images are omitted (Fig. 7.18) [59].

Another potential application of pancreatic spectral CT is dual-energy-based perfusion whereby the differences in perfusion, permeability, and blood volume between normal pancreatic parenchyma and tumors are assessed. One recent study [60] demonstrated that compared with single-energy CT, spectral perfusion CT permits a more accurate calculation of differences in perfusion, permeability, and blood volume between pancreatic tumors and healthy parenchyma. These authors speculated that the higher accuracy of spectral-based measurements is due to the use of linearly blended simulated 120-kVp images that are created with a combination of image data averaging 30 % from the low kVp and image data averaging 70 % from the high kVp. This technique combines the advantages of increased (iodine) contrast enhancement at 80 kVp with the low image noise at 140 kVp [60]. Spectral-based perfusion CT is a promising technique that needs further investigation.

By exploiting the attributes of improved tissue characterization over standard single-energy MDCT, spectral MDCT may provide a variety of advantages if implemented in routine pancreatic imaging. Imaging at lower energies can optimize the conspicuity of focal pancreatic lesions while achieving a significant radiation dose saving. Further advantages can be obtained by means of virtual unenhanced and iodine-only reconstructions.

Future perspectives for pancreatic imaging include the use of spectral-based iodine quantification and monochromatic imaging. Iodine quantification is a new approach that is independent of attenuation measurement while providing the iodine concentration in a lesion. Rather than a change in enhancement, this method depicts the presence and amount of iodine in a lesion, providing a more direct measure of tumor vascularity [61]. Monochromatic images are created by applying a mathematical model to the source data (polychromatic) obtained from scanning at two different energies [62, 63]. The images generated in this fashion mimic those that would be generated from a true monochromatic X-ray source having the same energy. Preliminary evidence [62, 63] suggests that compared to standard 120-kVp polychromatic images, monochromatic images are less susceptible to beam-hardening artifact and have the potential to provide more accurate and more reproducible attenuation measurements. Further research is needed to validate the accuracy and feasibility of spectral-based iodine quantification and monochromatic imaging before their use becomes widespread in pancreatic imaging.

References

1. Paspulati RM (2005) Multidetector CT of the pancreas. Radiol Clin North Am 43:999–1020
2. Lowenfels AB, Sullivan T, Fiorianti J, Maisonneuve P (2005) The epidemiology and impact of pancreatic diseases in the United States. Curr Gastroenterol Rep 7:90–95
3. Siegel R, Naishadham D, Jemal A (2012) Cancer statistics. CA Cancer J Clin 62:10–29
4. Hruban RH, Maitra A, Kern SE, Goggins M (2007) Precursors to pancreatic cancer. Gastroenterol Clin North Am 36:831–849
5. Megibow AJ (2010) Are we really closer to predicting the development of pancreatic cancer? Radiology 254:642–646
6. Klapman J, Malafa MP (2008) Early detection of pancreatic cancer: why, who, and how to screen. Cancer Control 15:280–287

7. Canto MI, Goggins M, Hruban RH et al (2006) Screening for early pancreatic neoplasia in high-risk individuals: a prospective controlled study. Clin Gastroenterol Hepatol 4:766–778
8. Bashir MR, Gupta RT (2012) MDCT evaluation of the pancreas: nuts and bolts. Radiol Clin North Am 50:365–377
9. Prokesch RW, Chow LC, Beaulieu CF, Bammer R, Jeffrey RB (2002) Isoattenuating pancreatic adenocarcinoma at multi-detector row CT: secondary signs. Radiology 224:764–768
10. Eaton SB Jr, Ferrucci JT Jr (eds) (1973) Radiology of the pancreas and duodenum. Saunders, Philadelphia
11. Haaga JR, Alfidi RJ, Zelch MG et al (1976) Computed tomography of the pancreas. Radiology 120:589–595
12. Stanley RJ, Sagel SS, Levitt RG (1977) Computed tomographic evaluation of the pancreas. Radiology 124:715–722
13. Gangi S, Fletcher JG, Nathan MA et al (2004) Time interval between abnormalities seen on CT and the clinical diagnosis of pancreatic cancer: retrospective review of CT scans obtained before diagnosis. AJR Am J Roentgenol 182:897–903
14. Hollett MD, Jorgensen MJ, Jeffrey RB (1995) Quantitative evaluation of pancreatic enhancement during dual-phase helical CT. Radiology 195:359–361
15. Tabuchi T, Itoh K, Ohshio G et al (1999) Tumor staging of pancreatic adenocarcinoma using early- and late-phase helical CT. AJR Am J Roentgenol 173:375–380
16. Keogan MT, McDermott VG, Paulson EK et al (1997) Pancreatic malignancy: effect of dual-phase helical CT in tumor detection and vascular opacification. Radiology 205:513–518
17. Graf O, Boland GW, Warshaw AL, Fernandez-del Castillo C, Hahn PF, Mueller PR (1997) Arterial versus portal venous helical CT for revealing pancreatic adenocarcinoma: conspicuity of tumor and critical vascular anatomy. AJR Am J Roentgenol 169:119–123
18. Lu DS, Vedantham S, Krasny RM, Kadell B, Berger WL, Reber HA (1996) Two-phase helical CT for pancreatic tumors: pancreatic versus hepatic phase enhancement of tumor, pancreas, and vascular structures. Radiology 199:697–701
19. Tanaka S, Nakao M, Ioka T et al (2010) Slight dilatation of the main pancreatic duct and presence of pancreatic cysts as predictive signs of pancreatic cancer: a prospective study. Radiology 254:965–972
20. Brennan DDD, Zamboni GA, Raptopoulos VD, Kruskal JB (2007) Comprehensive preoperative assessment of pancreatic adenocarcinoma with 64-section volumetric CT. Radiographics 27:1653–1666
21. Beger HG, Rau B, Gansauge F et al (2003) Treatment of pancreatic cancer: challenge of the facts. World J Surg 27:1075–1084
22. Ichikawa T, Ertuk SE, Sou H et al (2006) MDCT of pancreatic adenocarcinoma: optimal imaging phases and multiplanar reformatted imaging. AJR Am J Rentgenol 187:1513–1520
23. Kondo H, Kanematsu M, Goshima S et al (2007) MDCT of the pancreas: optimizing scanning delay with a bolus tracking technique for pancreatic, peripancreatic vascular, and hepatic contrast enhancement. AJR Am J Rentgenol 188:751–756
24. Freeny PC, Marks WM, Ryan JA, Traverso LW (1988) Pancreatic ductal adenocarcinoma: diagnosis and staging with dynamic CT. Radiology 166:125–133
25. Freeny PC (1989) Radiologic diagnosis and staging of pancreatic ductal adenocarcinoma. Radiol Clin North Am 27:121–128
26. Zeiss J, Coombs RJ, Bielke D (1990) CT presentation and staging accuracy of pancreatic adenocarcinoma. Int J Pancreatol 7:49–53
27. Dupuy DE, Costello P, Ecker CP (1992) Spiral CT of the pancreas. Radiology 183:815–818
28. Ichikawa T, Peterson MS, Federle MP et al (2000) Islet cell tumor of the pancreas: biphasic CT versus MR imaging in tumor detection. Radiology 216:163–171
29. Fletcher JG, Wiersema MJ, Farrell MA et al (2003) Pancreatic malignancy: value of arterial, pancreatic, and hepatic phase imaging with multi-detector row CT. Radiology 229:81–90
30. Choi BI, Chung MJ, Han JK, Han MC, Yoon YB (1997) Detection of pancreatic adenocarcinoma: relative value of arterial and late phases of spiral CT. Abdom Imaging 22:199–203
31. Boland GW, O'Malley ME, Saez M, Fernandez-del-Castillo C, Warshaw AL, Mueller PR (1999) Pancreatic-phase versus portal vein-phase helical CT of the pancreas: optimal temporal window for evaluation of pancreatic adenocarcinoma. AJR Am J Roentgenol 172:605–608
32. Nishiharu T, Yamashita Y, Ogata I et al (1998) Spiral CT of the pancreas. The value of small field-of-view targeted reconstruction. Acta Radiol 39:60–63
33. Horton KM, Fishman EK (2002) Multidetector CT angiography of pancreatic carcinoma: part 1, evaluation of arterial involvement. AJR Am J Roentgenol 178:827–831
34. Horton KM, Fishman EK (2000) 3D CT angiography of the celiac and superior mesenteric arteries with multidetector CT data sets: preliminary observations. Abdom Imaging 25:523–525
35. Novick SL, Fishman EK (1998) Three-dimensional CT angiography of pancreatic carcinoma: role in staging extent of disease. AJR Am J Roentgenol 170:139–143
36. Lu DSK, Reber HA, Krasny RM, Kadell BM, Sayre J (1997) Local staging of pancreatic cancer: criteria for unresectability of major vessels as revealed by pancreatic-phase, thin-section helical CT. AJR Am J Roentgenol 168:1439–1443
37. Horton KM, Fishman EK (2002) Multidetector CT angiography of pancreatic carcinoma: part 2, evaluation of venous involvement. AJR Am J Roentgenol 178:833–836

38. Fukushima H, Itoh S, Takada A et al (2006) Diagnostic value of curved multiplanar reformatted images in multislice CT for the detection of resectable pancreatic ductal adenocarcinoma. Eur Radiol 16:1709–1718
39. Hong KC, Freeny PC (1999) Pancreaticoduodenal arcades and dorsal pancreatic artery: comparison of CT angiography with three-dimensional volume rendering, maximum intensity projection, and shaded-surface display. AJR Am J Roentgenol 172:925–931
40. Bluemke DA, Cameron JL, Hruban RH et al (1995) Potentially resectable pancreatic adenocarcinoma: spiral CT assessment with surgical and pathologic correlation. Radiology 197:381–385
41. Diehl SJ, Lehmann KJ, Sadick M et al (1998) Pancreatic cancer: value of dual-phase helical CT in assessing resectability. Radiology 206:373–378
42. Valls C, Andia E, Sanchez A et al (2002) Dual-phase helical CT of pancreatic adenocarcinoma: assessment of resectability before surgery. AJR Am J Roentgenol 178:821–826
43. Roche CJ, Hughes ML, Garvey CJ et al (2003) CT and pathologic assessment of prospective nodal staging in patients with ductal adenocarcinoma of the head of the pancreas. AJR Am J Roentgenol 180:475–480
44. Imbriaco M, Megibow AJ, Ragozzino A et al (2005) Value of the single-phase technique in MDCT assessment of pancreatic tumors. AJR Am J Roentgenol 184:1111–1117
45. Imbriaco M, Megibow AJ, Camera L et al (2002) Dual-phase versus single-phase helical CT to detect and assess resectability of pancreatic carcinoma. AJR Am J Roentgenol 178:1473–1479
46. Marin D, Nelson RC, Barnhart H et al (2010) Detection of pancreatic tumors, image quality, and radiation dose during the pancreatic parenchymal phase: effect of a low-tube-voltage, high-tube-current ct technique—preliminary results. Radiology 256:450–459
47. Schindera ST, Nelson RC, Mukundan S Jr et al (2008) Hypervascular liver tumors: low tube voltage, high tube current multi-detector row CT for enhanced detection—phantom study. Radiology 246:125–132
48. Marin D, Nelson RC, Samei E et al (2009) Hypervascular liver tumors: low tube voltage, high tube current multidetector CT during late hepatic arterial phase for detection—initial clinical experience. Radiology 251:771–779
49. Schindera ST, Diedrichsen L, Muller HC et al (2011) Iterative reconstruction algorithm for abdominal multidetector CT at different tube voltages: assessment of diagnostic accuracy, image quality, and radiation dose in a phantom study. Radiology 260:454–462
50. Singh S, Kalra MK, Hsieh J et al (2010) Abdominal CT: comparison of adaptive statistical iterative and filtered back projection reconstruction techniques. Radiology 257:373–383
51. Marin D, Nelson RC, Schindera ST et al (2010) Low-tube-voltage, high-tube-current multidetector abdominal CT: improved image quality and decreased radiation dose with adaptive statistical iterative reconstruction algorithm—initial clinical experience. Radiology 254:145–153
52. Macari M, Spieler B, Kim D (2010) Dual-source dual-energy MDCT of pancreatic adenocarcinoma: initial observations with data generated at 80 kVp and at simulated weighted-average 120 kVp. AJR Am J Roentgenol 194:W27–W32
53. Johnson TR, Krauss B, Sedlmair M et al (2007) Material differentiation by dual energy CT: initial experience. Eur Radiol 17:1510–1517
54. Wintersperger B, Jakobs T, Herzog P et al (2005) Aorto-iliac multidetector-row CT angiography with low kV settings: improved vessel enhancement and simultaneous reduction of radiation dose. Eur Radiol 15:334–341
55. Patel BN, Thomas JV, Lockhart ME, Berland LL, Morgan DE (2013) Single-source dual-energy spectral multidetector CT of pancreatic adenocarcinoma: optimization of energy level viewing significantly increases lesion contrast. Clin Radiol 68:148–154
56. Heye T, Nelson RC, Ho LM, Marin D, Boll DT (2012) Dual-energy CT applications in the abdomen. AJR Am J Roentgenol 199:S64–S70
57. Graser A, Johnson TRC, Chandarana H, Macari M (2009) Dual energy CT: preliminary observations and potential clinical applications in the abdomen. Eur Radiol 19:13–23
58. Chu AJ, Lee JM, Lee YJ, Moon SK, Han JK, Choi BI (2012) Dual-source, dual-energy multidetector CT for the evaluation of pancreatic tumours. Br J Radiol 85:e891–e898
59. Mileto A, Mazziotti S, Gaeta M et al (2012) Pancreatic dual-source dual-energy CT: is it time to discard unenhanced imaging? Clin Radiol 67:334–339
60. Klauss M, Stillera W, Pahna G et al (2013) Dual-energy perfusion-CT of pancreatic adenocarcinoma. Eur J Radiol 82:208–214
61. Chandarana H, Megibow AJ, Cohen BA et al (2011) Iodine quantification with dual-energy CT: phantom study and preliminary experience with renal masses. AJR Am J Roentgenol 196:W693–W700
62. Yu L, Leng S, McCollough CH (2012) Dual-energy CT–based monochromatic imaging. AJR Am J Roentgenol 199:S9–S15
63. Silva AC, Morse BG, Hara AK, Paden RG, Hongo N, Pavlicek W (2011) Dual-energy (spectral) CT: applications in abdominal imaging. Radiographics 31:1031–1046

Index

G. Ascenti et al., *CT of the Retroperitoneum*,
DOI: 10.1007/978-88-470-5469-1, © Springer-Verlag Italia 2014

MIX
Papier aus verantwortungsvollen Quellen
Paper from responsible sources
FSC® C105338

If you have any concerns about our products,
you can contact us on
ProductSafety@springernature.com

In case Publisher is established outside the EU,
the EU authorized representative is:
Springer Nature Customer Service Center GmbH
Europaplatz 3, 69115 Heidelberg, Germany

Printed by Libri Plureos GmbH
in Hamburg, Germany